Praise for *Bodytypology*

"Anyone who is struggling with their food choices and weight needs to stop what they are doing and read this now. In her book, Sue-Anne does a great job explaining what might be holding you back from your goals and giving you concrete, easy-to-follow steps to get you on track for your body type. Having put her advice into practice, I've benefited by losing over 20 pounds, and now feel more energetic, positive, and have fewer body aches overall."

—Laura Lewis Hammond

"With clarity and thoughtful practicality, Sue-Anne details *Bodytypology* and invites the reader on a holistic journey of self-reflection and discovery. This journey to enhanced health and a balanced lifestyle is reinforced with motivational examples and tools readily available to the reader. Thank you, Sue-Anne, for sharing your insights, passion, and commitment to promoting the health of others. Well done!"

—Shari Mayer Gagné, Former Healthcare Professional

"Sue-Anne Hickey's *Bodytypology: A System for Optimal Health and Weight Loss* has been a revelation for me. This book has fundamentally changed my understanding of how my body and personality influence my dietary needs. Incorporating more protein and complex carbs has created a noticeable difference in my energy levels throughout the day. Bodytypology has provided me with a personalized approach to health that feels both intuitive and effective."

—Jenn Walker

"Reading *Bodytypology* has been a wonderful journey. In 2018 Sue-Anne helped me lose weight with her method and I also experienced a whole new awareness about my mind-body connection.

I was so happy to dive into *Bodytypology* all over again with her new book, highly recommend."

—Ana María Giraldo Ramirez, M.D.

"If you're tired of one-size-fits-all weight loss advice and are ready for a refreshing perspective, look no further than *Bodytypology* by Sue-Anne Hickey. This book is a game-changer, offering not only practical strategies for losing weight but also a deep dive into the concept of body types and how they influence weight loss success.

What sets this book apart is the author offers personalized recommendations based on your body type, ensuring that you're fueling your body with the right foods for optimal results. This will revolutionize the way you think about weight loss—and maybe even change your life."

—Debora Must, Spiritual Advisor

"As an active mom and a fitness coach, staying fit and eating well is an important focus for me. However, after reading Sue-Anne's insightful book on *Bodytypology*, I discovered several areas where I could make specific improvements to what and when I eat, to benefit my mood and energy levels while working toward weight and training goals. Thank you, Sue-Anne, for your dedication to promoting a sustainable approach to health and well-being!"

—Jennie Whitaker, CrossFit Trainer

"Sue-Anne is truly passionate about health and wellness. *Bodytypology* is just one of the ways she's made it her life's work to share valuable information and tips about how eating right for your body type can help you live your healthiest and best life. Sue-Anne is an authentic and beautiful inspiration to us all."

—Renee Mollitt, Yoga Instructor

"This book is a classic reference book; I loved the way it was organized, efficient, and offered me personalized suggestions and recipes, as if I had my own personal coach right there beside me. A wonderfully concise guide to taking care of yourself."

—Dr. Joanna McDonald, DM

"Sue-Anne Hickey acknowledges that we are all different and translates that concept into practical steps for healthier living.

Bodytypology is not just a book but a comprehensive guide. It provides a deep understanding of how our body functions, and valuable tips and recipes, making it a must-have health manual."

—Arantza Izurrategui

"The clarity Sue-Anne uses to explain the different body types is so helpful in determining your type. She gives many great healthy eating tips as well! For those of us who have tried many other restrictive diet programs, this is such a positive, sustainable way to eat healthily.

I also love the simple and easy, fabulous recipes. *Bodytypology* is such a helpful and informative book on eating well!"

—Melanie Cleland

"If you're looking for a breakthrough in your weight loss journey, this book is a game-changer. With its well-researched, concise approach, it dives deep into the crucial connection between body types and weight loss. This insightful guide will help you uncover the hidden barriers that have hindered your progress in the past, offering personalized strategies that align with your unique physiology.

Whether you're struggling to shed those last few pounds or embarking on a major health transformation, this book equips you with the knowledge and tools to regain control of your health and achieve sustainable weight loss. An essential read for anyone serious about understanding their body and unlocking their true potential."

—Valerie Provost

"Sue-Anne's book unlocks the unique differences hidden in our metabolism in her Bodytypology System. This system explains a new way to restore health and lose excess weight with simple changes to diet and lifestyle and inspiring stories of her client's transformations. These guidelines help the reader avoid hidden pitfalls found in following standard nutritional advice.

Her book explains the complex dynamics of nutrition, functional medicine, emotional trauma, hormones, and detoxification. A must-read for those who are seeking a new way to overcome their struggles with weight gain or loss, fatigue, and chronic pain."

—Greg Lee, Founder of the Lyme Research & Healing Center

BODY TYPOLOGY

A System for **Optimal Health** and Weight Loss

SUE-ANNE HICKEY

For Phil... I love you with all my heart.

Table of Contents

Introduction

When people want to lose weight or eat healthier, they look for a diet plan on the assumption that what works for others will for them too. Unfortunately, that's not how your body functions. You might lose weight but end up feeling tired and irritable. Or you might feel okay but gain weight.

The problem is that most people are unaware of their body's metabolism and specific needs. Bodytypology changes all of that!

In this system there are four body types, dictated by the gland that tends to be an 'overworker' in each type: Gonad, Adrenal, Thyroid and Pituitary. Each type has a different metabolism. People who want to lose weight must first understand their particular body type and then adapt to its unique rhythm to successfully reach their ideal weight and peak health.

Remember the old adage: "Eat breakfast like a king, lunch like a prince, and dinner like a pauper?"

If you are an Adrenal Type or Gonad Type in the Bodytypology system, you have a metabolism that is slowest in the morning. So this advice results in weight gain and may even cause you to feel hungry and eat more all day long. Nothing could be worse! You'd be much better off with a light breakfast, a medium to light lunch, and then dinner as the main meal of the day. This way, you can enjoy your most consistent meal when your metabolism is working fastest, and you will burn off that food.

If you are a Pituitary Type, the proverb suits you as a light vegetarian dinner is best for you, but the Thyroid Type needs three high-protein meals to keep feeling full and energetic all day.

When I started my naturopathy studies, I discovered I was a Thyroid Type. Over the next few months, I swapped my breakfast cereal for two eggs, decreased my bread intake and increased my protein at lunch and dinner. I learned to better manage my stress by cycling more and took supplements and vitamins to balance my nutritional deficiencies.

The change was spectacular! My ghost-like complexion took on a healthy glow, I wasn't constantly reaching for carbs or sweets anymore, and I went from being one of the slowest members in my large, urban cycling club to one of the fastest women. Learning to eat right for my body type is the single most beneficial thing I ever did to transform my health and my life.

When I started working as a naturopath, I was sharing the program with clients to help improve their overall health — weight loss was a side-benefit.

But word of mouth quickly made me known as a weight loss specialist because my clients were not only losing weight but keeping it off and, most importantly, feeling healthier and more energetic. I continue to have a steady influx of clients for this reason.

To help as many people as possible, this book was born. While the focus is primarily to help those who want to improve their overall health or lose weight, I believe that we all greatly benefit by learning how to eat right for our specific body type. By following my suggestions for healthy eating, you'll likely see your strength and stamina improve, your specific cravings and mood swings reduce, and unwanted pounds disappear in the process. All without going hungry or being undernourished.

Nearly all the clients who come to see me say that they have already tried everything. Some even use the word *desperate*.

Why does one person thrive on a certain diet while another feels awful? Why do some people lose weight easily, while others struggle? How is it that one individual will gain weight in the stomach area, but another gains on the buttocks or thighs? What accounts for people's diverse cravings?

We're all different!

Too many people are depriving themselves of their favorite foods, counting calories or points, trying and then dropping the latest fad diets, and losing weight only to gain it all back. It's essential to stop the yo-yo dieting. This will cause your metabolism to slow, which in turn leads to more weight gain in the future.

A healthy eating plan must be personalized to each individual's metabolism, energy levels, cravings, body shape, and glandular imbalances. Not only for weight loss but for optimal health, strength, endurance and high energy.

Sophia contacted me after blood tests showed her C reactive protein and some liver enzymes were high, indicating chronic or systemic inflammation in the body. She followed her Gonad Type plan as well, replacing wheat with Kamut Khorasan wheat or spelt and reducing sugar and dairy. Four months later, her blood test results showed her C reactive protein and liver enzymes were normal and she was happy to have dropped 11 pounds.

Tom was an Adrenal Type who was prone to frequent headaches, as well as having high cholesterol and high triglycerides. At 55, he wanted to be in better physical shape and to lead the second part of his life much healthier than that first half. By eating right for his body type as well as reducing his alcohol intake and increasing water, he had much more energy, his afternoon energy slumps were gone, and he lost 27 pounds in 12 weeks. A few months later, his blood test showed a great improvement overall.

If you determine your body type and follow the plan outlined here, you will lose excess weight over a relatively short period of time, keep it off, and, most importantly, transform your health and life!

This book provides you with guidelines specifically for your body type. It will show you the kinds of food you need to eat and when. It will also suggest healthier alternatives to your current cravings. It will recommend the best kinds of exercise for your body type, and the most beneficial vitamins, supplements, and herbal teas.

Everyone indulges in a special meal or dessert once in a while. But if you are having a hard time sticking with your body type's plan, there may be some underlying reasons. Based on my experience with clients, these often go back to our childhood. That's why I have included a section on emotional eating where I share my own past efforts to stuff down my feelings in unhealthy ways.

Okay, let's get started!

Part One

What is Bodytypology and What's in it for Me?

Who Can Benefit from Eating Healthily for Their Body Type?

Actually, everyone! However, let's start with specific groups who've been particularly stuck. After over a decade of working with clients, I've noticed they tend to fall into one of the following groups...

Those Who Want to Lose Weight and Have Tried Other Ways

You've tried other diets, but they haven't worked. They left you feeling hungry, moody, perhaps downright irritable. You've deprived yourself of your favorite foods, had very little energy, and felt discouraged, even defeated.

I will emphasize up front: this is not a rapid weight loss program. When I start working with clients, one of the first questions is often: "How fast will I lose the weight?"

We live in an age of immediate gratification, always seeking ways to speed things up. Rapid weight loss is a product of this culture. Bottom line: it's unhealthy.

And there is no norm. Everybody — by which I really mean every *body* — has a unique experience. Some will lose more quickly in the first week;

others will take more time for the weight loss to start. The more closely you follow your body type's plan and the more you move your body in ways it will best respond, the more quickly the pounds will likely drop. Most of my clients lose one to two pounds a week until they reach their desired goal. Then they keep on with the lifestyle to maintain a healthy weight.

The most important thing I want to teach my clients is to learn to eat healthily in a way they can easily sustain on their own for the rest of their lives.

This is primarily about regaining your health with the ideal eating regimen and lifestyle for your body type. The weight loss will happen naturally. By eating right for your body type, you will also change your body shape. Bodytypology will help to dissolve weight from the places where you most want it gone.

Those Who Want to Enjoy Balanced Energy All Day Every Day

Aside from weight loss, there is another most common request that comes from new clients. They want to increase their energy.

If you wake up tired and take a long time to get going... If you have up and down energy all day... If your energy slumps after meals, or in the afternoon... If you need coffee or sweets to make it through the day... If your energy is never very high... this book is for you.

It is not normal to always have low energy or feel tired. Our natural birthright is to have abundant energy throughout the day so we can enjoy all of life's possibilities. By following your plan, your energy will increase enormously.

Those Who Have Difficulty with Cravings

Each time I ask my clients what their biggest cravings are, I get completely different responses. Everything from sugar pie to liver with onions to chips is mentioned. This goes to show that different people need different dietary plans.

Cravings often indicate a nutritional deficiency and/or a need to suppress negative feelings. By nourishing your body with certain healthy foods at the right time, your cravings will diminish and ultimately disappear. You will also become keenly aware of any emotional eating patterns and do something healthier to manage your feelings instead. (I have some wonderfully effective suggestions for you and you can download a free Emotional Eating Food Journal at https://www.bodytypology.com/book.html.)

If your downfall is chocolate or other kinds of sweets, there is a plan for you. If you can't stay away from chips and other salty foods, there is a plan for you. Some people yearn for creamy sauces, while still others crave fried or fatty food. Whatever your cravings, this book will help you to keep them in check.

Vegans and Vegetarians

I was a vegetarian for 16 years and I believe that a plant-based diet is the healthiest diet that we can eat. When I was vegetarian, people often asked me how I managed to consume enough protein. I would become rather irate, exclaiming, "There's protein in everything!" While that may be true, many vegetables and fruit contain only minimal amounts of protein. When I took my classes to become a naturopath, I learned the importance of adequate protein in a diet and how to ensure I was getting enough for my body type. More specifically, I learned that I was deficient in vitamin B12 and iron.

Bodytypology works for vegans and vegetarians. (Gonad and Adrenal types especially thrive on a plant-based diet.) It is important to educate yourself or consult with a specialist when following a vegetarian or vegan diet to ensure all your nutritional requirements are being met. There are now also apps such as MyFitnessPal or MyPlate to help ensure you're getting enough protein.

Athletes

Perhaps you don't need to lose weight but want to increase your strength and stamina. You eat what you consider to be a healthy diet, but you want to know what else your body needs to surpass your personal best at your sport.

I joined a cycling club at the same time as I started my naturopath classes. On our initial rides, I would peddle and coast, peddle and coast. I was constantly increasing and decreasing my speed. This creates a problem because one of the main goals in a group of cyclists is to maintain a steady pace. An older club member rode up alongside me and asked me to try to pedal more steadily. "I can't," I replied. "I get too tired." At the end of the approximately 25-mile ride, I would collapse onto the couch, unable to move for the rest of the day.

Over the next couple of years, as I implemented what I'd learned about my body type's plan, I became the only female rider most often in a group of 12 to 14 men, most of whom were racers. After 60-mile or longer rides at a fast pace, I would get on with my day, even clean my house, as if it were nothing. Maybe cycling isn't your thing, but implementing your plan will give you the strength and stamina to do all your physical activities with greater ease.

Those Who Feel Tired or Lack Motivation

You believe you are eating healthily but you know something is off. You never feel your energy is a ten out of ten. There are also those last few pounds that always seem impossible to lose. Perhaps ever since you've had children it's been more difficult to get back to the level of health you enjoyed beforehand, that feeling of balance and positivity you previously had. Following your plan will help you to regain the health, energy, and balance to help you feel happier again.

Those With Ailments, Allergies or Illnesses

One of the best things you can do to improve your overall health is to follow your body type's plan. It might strengthen your immune system and increase your body's natural ability to heal. After I started implementing everything I was learning as a naturopath for my body type, my blood sugar levels normalized and the eczema I had for 20 years disappeared forever. I felt energized and better than ever.

Before doing an initial consultation with my clients, I send them a health history form to fill out and return to me. After working with them for three to six months, we go back over their health history form and often they are surprised as, invariably, issues such as bloating, acid reflux, indigestion, headaches, or PMS challenges have greatly diminished or disappeared. Often, their blood tests also indicate significant improvement.

Take, for example, this testimonial from a Gonad-Type client of mine.

"I was hoping Sue-Anne could help me with four issues: digestion, which was my main ailment, along with poor sleep, joint pain, and my weight. My digestion improved tremendously in only ten days, and I was sleeping better. Within the next month, the pain in my joints (shoulders, elbows, hips, and knees) subsided. And, bonus, I was losing weight!

"Three months later, my digestive issues are gone! I sleep soundly for eight hours every night, I have hardly any pain left in my joints, and I've lost 12 pounds! The knowledge will stay with me forever. Eating for my body type has changed my life! It is simple, easy to follow, and it works."

Of course, I always tell my clients to seek the proper medical advice for their ailments. And eating right for your body type helps with healing, too. I've had hundreds of clients report their health issues have become less severe or disappeared entirely.

What Can I Expect When I Follow My Personal Plan?

Easily Lose Weight in the Areas Where You Most Want to Do So

"Why do I always gain weight there?" clients lament, especially those who tend to gain on the lower body. Your Bodytypology plan will help the weight come off, no matter where it is. You will also learn what exercises are best suited for your body type to help you slim down where desired.

Increase and Balance Your Energy

Some body types fare better in the morning, some are more productive and do their best work later in the day. No matter what your type, your energy will be more stable. You won't experience crashes after meals or mid-afternoon; nor will you need as many stimulants, such as coffee or sweets, to keep you going.

I had a client who was 71 years old and had always felt guilty because she needed a lot of sleep. Imagine her relief when I told her that was normal for her Gonad body type!

By figuring out your own energy levels, you will be able to understand your body's own natural rhythms and adjust your lifestyle.

Cut Cravings and Feel Completely Satisfied, Not Hungry

Many people that want to lose weight think they must deprive themselves. Nothing could be further from the truth. One of the comments I hear most often from my clients is, "This is easy. I don't feel hungry."

It's the refined and processed foods that have you feeling hungry soon after. With the right nutritious food for your body type, your cravings will be a thing of the past.

Nutritionally dense foods will keep you feeling full.

Increase Your Strength and Endurance

Members of my cycling club always wanted to know what I did to get so much stronger and faster, even as I aged. By following my plan and listening to my body, I feed myself what I need to maintain my health, strength and endurance. You can also enjoy these results.

Gain Overall Well-Being

When you nourish your body and balance your glands with the right food for you, your body becomes more stable. As a result, you will feel calmer overall. Your cheeks will also be rosier as you take on a healthier glow inside and out.

A Plan That Works for You Long-Term

There are too many diets that are overly restrictive, making them impossible to follow for any real length of time. Most people regain any weight they've lost and often find it harder to lose the second time. This book will provide you with a plan you can easily follow for the rest of your life.

Where Did This System Come From?

It was a warm fall day in 2006 when I asked a friend to meet me for lunch at one of Montreal's trendy Plateau neighborhood cafés. I was a self-employed yoga teacher and wanted to learn more about the classes she had taken to become a naturopath. While we talked and munched on our sandwiches, it soon became clear to me naturopathy would be something I'd love to do. I drove home, emailed the teacher, and found out that the fall session would start that Saturday! I showed up at 8:30 a.m., check in hand, not realizing that I was embarking on part-time studies that would last six years and lead me to my calling.

I was fortunate to study under Lise Harbeck, a naturopath with degrees in chemistry and nutrition and more than twenty years of experience.

The first thing we studied was the body-type plan. It's originator, Dr. Henry Bieler (1839-1975,) was well known for his book, *Food is Your Best Medicine*. He was a physician and a nutritionist who introduced the concept of distinguishing individuals by identifying their dominant gland. He determined there were Thyroid Types and Adrenal Types and that these dominant glands affected the shape of a person's body. Thyroid Types are more often tall and slender, while Adrenal Types are usually stockier. He believed there was also a third type, but never fully worked it out.

In 1983, Dr. Elliot Abravanel co-authored the book, *Dr. Abravanel's Body Type Diet and Lifetime Nutrition Plan*. Inspired by Bieler's theory, Abravanel determined two more types with his own research: the Gonad Type (among women only, despite the name's male connotations) and the Pituitary Type. He discovered a direct link between each of these types and where fat accumulated on a person's body. When he put two of his patients on the same weight loss plan, one lost weight and felt great, while the other lost very little weight, became pale, felt tired, and experienced increased food cravings.

He realized the differences arose from the fact that different people have different metabolisms, energy levels, cravings, and dominant glands affecting their bodies. This doesn't mean that there is something wrong with the dominant gland, but simply that it is working harder than the others. The other glands are trying to catch up, and this creates an imbalance. He determined that the issue wasn't a certain diet per se, but rather the way each person's specific glands, metabolism and body type react to an eating plan. When he created different plans for different glandular types, suggesting different types of food to eat or avoid at specific times, his patients lost weight where they wanted to get rid of it and kept it off. Their health improved and their energy increased.

My teacher, Lise Harbeck, recognized the body-type plan as revolutionary and devised even healthier eating plans for each type. She found better alternatives for the diet mayonnaise, diet salad dressings, refined vegetable oils, cheeses, white sugar, and other less healthy options of decades past in the outdated guides.

She discovered that people who have diabetes or a tendency towards hypoglycemia fared better by following the Thyroid Type plan until their blood sugar levels were properly rebalanced before switching to their particular body type's plan.

My own life was transformed by following my body type's plan, so it became a focal point of my practice from the beginning. Although my original aim was to help people with their overall health, I quickly became known as a weight loss expert because of my clients' success in this area.

As I worked with clients, I began to understand more about how to support the emotional challenges each of the types faces. For instance, how the Gonad Type needs extra support to take care of herself and how the Adrenal type does well with a Complex B vitamin to help nourish their nervous system because they tend to internalize their stress. In this way, I developed my own signature program. While brainstorming names with a good friend, she came up with Bodytypology, which was (and still is) a perfect fit.

How Do I Determine My Body Type?

In my naturopathic classes, we learned there are two "salty" types and two "sweet" types. Adrenal and Gonad Body Types are "salty" types, as they generally crave salty food.

"Salty" Types

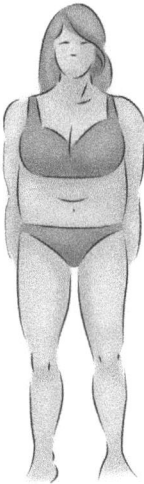 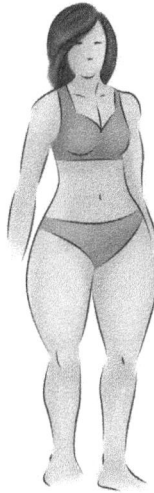 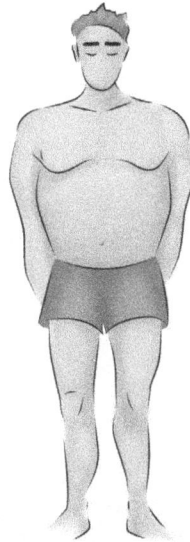

Adrenal   Gonad   Adrenal

Pituitary and Thyroid Types are "sweet" types as they tend to crave sweets or carbs.

"Sweet" Types

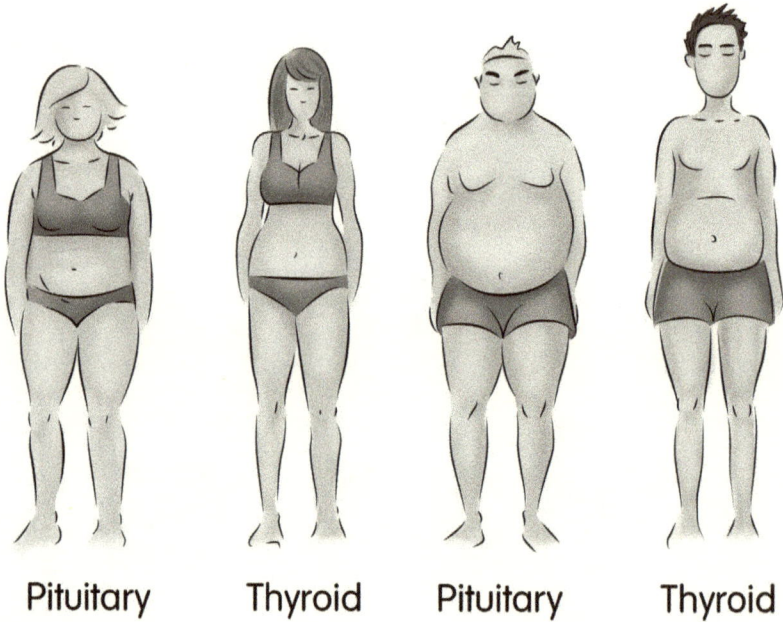

| Pituitary | Thyroid | Pituitary | Thyroid |

Adrenal Types may crave both salty and sweet food, although the sweets they enjoy tend to be richer, fattier desserts such as crème brûlée or pecan pie rather than hard candies. While an Adrenal Type will seek out chips for a hit of salt, Thyroid Types tend to seek out the same bag of chips for the carbohydrates.

Personal food preferences can lead to quite a bit of overlap in cravings among body types, so I often need to play the detective during client consultations to determine a person's body type. I'm sharing many of these clues with you to help you do your own detective work.

The areas where you tend to gain weight can be an indication of your type, but you can't determine your type by physical appearance alone. Most people are used to seeing pictures of different body shapes and trying to determine which type they are. It's important to note that with Bodytypology, there are many other factors to consider.

Most of the clients I see for weight loss are either Adrenal or Gonad Types.

Chances are, if you want to lose weight, you are one of the two "salty" types. Focus on the descriptions in the "salty" category to determine your body type.

Thyroid Types are generally tall, slim and don't tend to gain weight. If they do, it tends to be around the midsection.

You may think you resemble a Pituitary Type, gaining weight evenly, but think back to when you originally started to gain weight. Was it more in the upper body, like the Adrenal Type, or lower body like the Gonad Type? There are very few Pituitary Types, just five percent of the population and most of them are men.

The other main elements I assess when determining body type are as follows:

Energy Level

Are you a morning person? Do you jump out of bed ready to take on the day, or does it take you a while to get going? Do you have steady energy all day long or does your energy dip mid-afternoon? Some Adrenal or Gonad Types may be up at the crack of dawn, busy with getting the kids off to school and getting to work, so they may tell me they are a morning person, which may be true. However, given the choice on weekends, they prefer to start off their day at a slower pace, having some quiet time while enjoying their coffee. For that reason, the "salty" types are not really known as morning types as much as the "sweet" types. The "sweet" types are usually in high gear early. If a person can easily stay up until 11 PM or midnight, they probably are not a "sweet" type, for whom "early to bed, early to rise" suits best.

Food Preferences

Start with determining whether you're in the "salty" or "sweet" cravings camp.

Hunger Timing/Patterns

How hungry are you at different times of the day? If a client tells me they're not hungry in the morning and can go until 10 or 11 AM without eating, I can rule out the "sweet" types, which need to eat early.

Personality

One fascinating thing about Bodytypology is that the personality description often accurately reveals a person's body type. The Pituitary Type can tend to be introverted and known as the quiet thinking type, while many Adrenal Types love to socialize. Sometimes it's hard to see ourselves. I encourage you to read the full personality description of each type. If you've then narrowed your type down to two possibilities but are still having trouble figuring out exactly which one, have a good friend or your partner read the personality descriptions to see if they can help you to identify yours.

Ailments to Which You Are Prone

The Gonad Type is more susceptible to imbalances related to the ovaries so tend to have more ailments involving the reproductive system, such as breast or ovarian cysts, endometriosis, PMS challenges or menopause issues. Adrenal Types tend to have high blood pressure, high cholesterol, or a skin condition such as psoriasis. The Thyroid Type is prone to hypoglycemia or diabetes and their nervous energy can cause digestive problems. Pituitary Types may be prone to respiratory congestion, sinusitis and excess mucus due to consuming too much dairy.

Keep a Journal

I have new clients send me a three-day food and drink journal before I meet with them. Then I ask them to write down their existing ailments pertaining to each of their body's systems (digestive, respiratory, immune, etc.), and rate the frequency of their symptoms as: 1. Sometimes, 2. Often, or 3. Nearly always.

The journal often yields our answer, but sometimes it takes more digging into a person's lifestyle and food preferences.

Lisa told me she wanted to lose 40 to 50 pounds. She checked off very few ailments in her health history: only hot flashes and some minor digestive issues. She indicated her cholesterol was slightly high, so I thought she may be an Adrenal type. However, she was an investment advisor with three children. Gonad types are usually motherly, care-giving individuals. Often, they have three or four children. Lisa's career choice was not typical of a Gonad Type, who typically choose a career in the healing professions. But, as a financial advisor, she was taking care of her clients.

I asked her, "If you could eat anything at all, what would you grab?"

"A hamburger, French fries and fish," Lisa replied.

When I asked her preferences when it came to pasta sauce and salad dressing, she immediately said: "Meat sauce, and oil and vinegar."

These are the kind of answers an Adrenal Type would give.

The Gonad Type might choose French fries, as they do gravitate towards fried or salty food. Their pasta choices might be an Alfredo or rosé sauce and they might prefer Cesar or a creamy salad dressing.

I asked Lisa whether her face turned red when she exercised (an Adrenal trait).

She said, "No."

She then told me she tended to gain weight in her upper belly. This strongly pointed to her being an Adrenal Type.

We were communicating on Zoom. When I asked her to stand up and step back, I saw that her lower body and hips were larger than her upper body. Her chest was relatively small, indicating a Gonad Type.

Another important indicator of Gonad Types is whether they have cellulite. Gonad Types typically say they've had cellulite since their teens, while Adrenal Types may have only had it starting in their thirties or later, or not at all.

Lisa said she "always" had cellulite.

Another key clue is a person's preferred meal and snack times. When I suggested that Lisa might be ready to eat dinner at 5 PM, she agreed, which again indicated she was a Gonad Type. Adrenal Types might be able to delay eating dinner until 7 PM, no problem.

Gonad Types generally venture into the fridge or pantry late at night or during the wee hours of the morning, while Adrenal Types are more often afternoon snackers.

In going over Lisa's journal with her, I was able to determine that she was energetic in the morning simply because she rushed to get her kids ready for school without eating any breakfast herself. This is another indication of a Gonad Type because they will often take care of others to their own detriment. I asked her if she enjoyed the taste of peanut butter and toast and, like many Gonad Types, she said yes.

I often ask clients if it was important to them to have children. While most types will say yes, this is especially true for Gonad Types, and they often tell me that they breastfed their children for as long as was possible.

Of course, there are many Gonad Types who don't have children, but they often will be devoted to their work, pets, family, or friends.

Lisa was definitely a Gonad Type.

If, after reading descriptions of all the body types you're still not sure which type you are, you can take the Body Type Quiz:

https://www.bodytypology.com/book.html

What Plan Should Children Follow?

Growing children need a lot of protein, so they should follow the Thyroid Type plan until puberty, when they should be assessed. After puberty, a body type seldom changes, although occasionally it can happen after giving birth.

What Can I Do for My Health (Regardless of My Type)?

"I was so hungry yesterday!" some of my clients occasionally exclaim. When I ask them what they had for lunch or dinner the previous day, they often realize they had forgotten to eat enough protein or healthy carbohydrates. They had something like a Cesar salad for dinner, or a vegetable soup for lunch. Many people either don't know or forget that every meal plays into the next. A lack of protein and/or healthy carbohydrates will cause hunger during the day and even the following one.

Not every body type needs protein for breakfast, but everyone requires protein and healthy carbohydrates for lunch and dinner. Good protein sources include poultry, fish, any kind of beans such as chickpeas, lentils, black beans, tempeh, or tofu. Healthy carbohydrates include brown rice, quinoa, barley, sweet potatoes, and potatoes.

Aim to fill one quarter of your plate with protein, one quarter with healthy carbohydrates and the remaining half with vegetables. It may be challenging at first. Planning and preparing in advance is key. I often cook some quinoa while I'm having breakfast and then put the whole pot into the fridge so the quinoa cools down and is ready to be tossed in a salad for lunch. I make huge salads that last for days. I also freeze chili, soups, and casseroles for quick meals.

A Word on Dairy

If you are lactose-intolerant, it could indicate that you don't tolerate dairy at all and you might feel better without it altogether — even that little bit of cream in your coffee. For many people, dairy increases mucus production. This is the body's natural way of protecting itself from a substance it doesn't tolerate.

Whole Grains and Cereals

The Keto fad has given whole grains a bad rap by suggesting it's best to avoid all carbs. Whole grains are good for us. They are rich in B vitamins that nourish the nervous system and help to keep us calm. Whole grain products should be made with unrefined, unbleached flour that is preferably stone-ground to retain its nutritional benefits. A good choice for cereal is Nature's Path Kamut Khorasan Wheat Flakes. With only five grams of sugar, this cereal keeps many types satisfied until lunch. For other meals, choose whole grain brown rice, rye, buckwheat, quinoa, spelt, barley, millet, or Kamut Khorasan wheat over refined and bleached wheat.

I also prefer having pasta made from Kamut Khorasan wheat as it remains soft, and leftovers can be easily eaten cold in a pasta salad. Pasta made from whole grains or beans is good too. Brown rice pasta, less expensive than other kinds, must be cooked for the exact amount of required time. Undercooked, it will be hard, and it gets mushy if overdone. You may need to re-boil the leftovers to soften them again.

Non-cereals, such as potatoes and sweet potatoes, are nourishing and satiating carbs.

Herbal Teas

Each body type has specific herbal teas that are most beneficial. However, if you have any health conditions or are taking any prescribed medications, *always* consult with your doctor and pharmacist before drinking any herbal teas or taking any herbs. The wrong choice can exacerbate your condition or reduce the effectiveness of a medication. Once you've checked with your doctor or pharmacist, it is still wise to allow for two to three hours to pass between taking your medication and using any supplements, vitamins, herbs, or tea so they don't ever work at cross-purposes.

Herbal teas are not essential to drink, but they can provide beneficial nutrients and help you overcome cravings. For example, Thyroid Types often crave sweets that a raspberry leaf tea can satisfy. It's also an astringent herb that refreshes. Such a tea might also help a Thyroid Type to avoid stimulants like coffee (and the cream and sugar they might put in it).

Stress Management

Managing stress is vital for health and especially weight loss because stress signals the adrenal glands to secrete cortisol, which signals the body to retain weight for protection.

Sometimes when I ask my clients how they manage their stress, they respond by saying things such as, "I yell at my kids", "I drink", or "I eat. Why do you think I hired you?"

Joking aside, can you find better coping mechanisms when you suddenly feel like eating and it's not hunger? Deep abdominal breathing is one of the most effective, listening to soothing music, using essential oils, journaling, or whatever outlet helps you.

Detoxing Doesn't Have to Be Scary

When I taught yoga to beginners, some of them felt nauseated during their initial classes. The bending and twisting of some of the moves put pressure on some people's liver and internal organs, releasing toxins that caused nausea. Our bodies have many ways of naturally eliminating toxins through the liver, intestines, skin, lungs, and kidneys. However, it's important to occasionally help the body release excess toxins.

Some have the misconception that a detox will have them running to the bathroom all day, which is false. Others think they need to fast, depriving the body of essential nutrients. This unhealthy strategy guarantees you immediately regain any weight lost, and maybe some extra, during such a fast.

Our bodies are exposed to chemicals through air pollution, pesticides, herbicides, and additives in our food; as well as chemicals in cleaning products, skin care, flame retardant fabrics... the list goes on. It's important to do all we can to reduce our exposure to chemicals in our homes. You can find healthy alternatives in each of these areas.

I believe that exposure to toxins is one of the reasons why the incidence of cancer and other diseases is so high. The toxins in your body may also be the cause of your fatigue, headaches, or skin conditions. (Excess toxins are pushed out through the skin.) Our liver alone has more than 400 tasks to do. When menopausal women drink alcohol, their hot flashes increase — a sign the liver is overburdened and struggling to balance hormones at the same time.

Jessica had been enduring hot flashes for 13 years. She soaked the bedsheets every night with her sweat. She never wore long sleeves, never buttoned her coat, and never closed the windows in winter. She didn't want to use hormone replacement therapy as there was a history of hormonally dependent cancer in her family. With some changes to her diet and a single 30-day liver detox product I recommended, the hot flashes disappeared.

An occasional detox helps our liver to rid our body of toxins and keeps it functioning optimally in preparation for weight loss. A regular detox maintains a healthy, toxin-free body for continued weight loss. According to traditional Chinese medicine, spring is when internal energies rise and expand, making it a perfect time to detox. I recommend spring and fall as ideal times for a detox, although it can be done at any time.

A good quality natural detox can

- help the intestinal, digestive, and circulatory systems function better,
- restore the optimal function of weakened organs,
- provide a better assimilation of nutrients,
- promote the growth of friendly, digestive-aiding bacteria in the gut,
- strengthen the immune system, and
- support the liver's toxin-removing functions and the elimination of waste.

A good detox is simple. It involves taking some additional quality products and eating a healthy diet with plenty of fresh fruit and vegetables, especially dark leafy greens, and whole grains such as brown rice. It also involves drinking plenty of water while avoiding red meat, fried food, sugary food, coffee, and alcohol for a few weeks or a few months.

I sometimes suggest my clients use Nature's Sunshine products, as I find they are high-quality and reasonably priced. Dandelion capsules can be beneficial to all body types. Adrenal Types tend to have a congested liver so a 30-day detox I often recommend for them is Tiao He Cleanse in the U.S.

For the simplest liver detox, drink the freshly squeezed juice of half a lemon in a cup of hot water first thing in the morning. This helps the liver release toxins more effectively. If your teeth are sensitive to lemon, drink with a (stainless steel) straw.

The Importance of Fiber

During any other type of detox, you should have two to three bowel movements a day to avoid headaches or nausea and to ensure toxins are leaving your body. If you're not having regular bowel movements, then add extra fiber to your daily regime before you begin your detox. You can use freshly ground flax seeds or good quality aloe vera juice. Psyllium hulls or husks are another excellent option. These are a healthier alternative to laxatives that can make the colon lazy and compromise the natural peristaltic movement or wavelike action of the muscles that line your gastrointestinal tract. They simply add fiber to your diet and can even be taken long term if you're not regular. Avoid commercial brands of psyllium hulls that may be high in sugar, artificial flavors, and colors. Start with a small amount of fiber and gradually increase it as needed. If you choose to use flax seeds, ensure they are fresh. Whole flax seeds do not break down in the body, so you must grind them first. You can use a coffee or spice grinder. Once they are ground, keep them in the freezer as they can become rancid quickly.

Aloe vera juice is the easiest to take. It has a soothing effect on the digestive tract but is not as effective as psyllium hulls. Psyllium hulls have a similar effect as flax seed, and no grinding is necessary.

Psyllium hulls add bulk to your stool and increase the necessary transit time. Transit time, which is the time it takes food to get through the body, is normally 18 to 24 hours.

Start with one quarter-teaspoon in a full glass of water followed by a second full glass of water. After three days, increase to half a teaspoon and then keep increasing the amount gradually until you start having two to three bowel movements a day. For some, that may be a half teaspoon; for others, it may be one or two heaping tablespoons. Regardless of the amount, always take it with two full glasses of water. The amount of psyllium and water can be split to take at two different times during the day. It is rare, but some people have a long colon. If the psyllium stays too long in the colon, it increases transit time. In that case, aloe vera juice is a better alternative.

Once you're having two to three bowel movements daily, you're ready to start your detox. As one of the first wild plants to grow in the spring, dandelions are an invitation to cleanse the system after a long winter. High in potassium, dandelion is good for digestion and the liver. A dandelion supplement is an easy way to reap its benefits. They can be taken for six to eight weeks at a time.

Part Two

Everything You Wanted to Know About the Four Body Types

Gonad Type

Gonad Type: The Caregiver!
Time to Care for You

Despite its more common use as slang in reference to male genitals, a gonad refers to the organ containing the reproductive cells in both sexes — the testes in men and the ovaries in women. In the Bodytypology system, it's the ovaries that are the dominant gland, so *only women* can be Gonad Types.

Gonad Types tend to be the most giving people, sometimes to their own detriment.

Energy Levels

Gonad Types are more night owls than morning people, although many will be ready for bed by 9:30 or 10 PM. When balanced, they have stable energy that increases as the day progresses. Those who have low blood sugar (hypoglycemia) tend to experience an energy crash around 4 PM. (Anyone who has hypoglycemia, needs to follow the Thyroid Type plan until their sweet cravings are managed.) Some Thyroid Types get a second wind around

Sue-Anne Hickey

10 PM and can end up going to bed late, staying up, at times, until 2 AM. This is detrimental to their health. As Gonad Types need more sleep than any of the other types.

Gonad Types feel wonderful when they're able to get a good, long sleep on the weekend to refill a tank that can often be low on energy.

The Gonad body type is not typically as physically strong as others, but their energy tends to endure the longest. However, they need to go at their own, often slower, pace. Like the tortoise, when Gonad Types respect their bodies' natural rhythms, they often win the race!

Personality Traits: Home and Harmony

Some words that describe the Gonad Type: affectionate, emotional, attentive, kind, harmonious, ethical, empathetic, generous and altruistic. They have strong values, courage, and willpower.

Gonad Types are known for their warmth and love. Their strong maternal instincts distinguish them from the other types. About 75% of all nurses are Gonad Types. The other helping professions also tend to have high percentages of Gonad Types: social workers, teachers, massage therapists, psychologists, etc.

Being in a relationship is very important to Gonad Types, as is having children or pets. While a Thyroid Type can't wait to get out after having a baby, Gonad Types are in their glory at home, where they often breastfeed their children for a long time. They can actually be overly concerned for the welfare of their children and their tendency to do too much can become stifling for their kids. Because home and property are very important to Gonad Types they prefer not to travel for too long. When their children leave home, it is very hard on them.

Danielle wanted to increase her self-care time — a common struggle for Gonad Types. She made it one of her weekly goals to enjoy a leisurely bath. For two weeks she set this goal but then reported not having time. I suggested that she have a bath as soon as she arrived home from our meeting that evening. "Oh, no. I couldn't possibly do that," she exclaimed. "It's my son's birthday this weekend. I've rented a hall, we have a Ninja Turtle theme,

30

and I'm making all the decorations by hand."

This is a perfect example of the Gonad Type's generosity to the detriment of self.

If people who are this type don't have children, they may become overly devoted to work, or the care of their aging parents, or their pets. They also love to talk about life, to exchange views with others, and to share ideas. They can project 20 years into the future, no problem. When there is a conflict (which may be rare as they normally don't allow for conflict), they have a good sense of justice and search for ways to smooth things out.

Gonad Types are ill at ease with competition of any kind, as well as superficial or non-harmonious relationships. They also hate any sudden changes in 'the program', financial risk, or a lack of order.

They would do well to let people and things go, learn to live and let live, and think more about themselves and their self-care.

Physical Traits: Pear-Shaped

The Gonad Type may often exclaim, "Why do I always gain weight *there!*" '*There*' is the lower body, the sides of the upper thighs (also known as saddle bags), and the buttocks. They tend to be 'pear-shaped' with a larger lower body and a small to medium-sized upper body. Often, a Gonad Type's back slightly curves inward, making their buttocks more prominent. While other types may acquire cellulite later in life, Gonad Types tend to develop it at a young age. When I ask how long they've had cellulite, the answer nearly always is " forever!"

Common Ailments: Hormonal Imbalance

Typical problems relate to their reproductive organs or lymphatic system. This can include menstrual problems and/or premenstrual syndrome (PMS), mastitis, infertility, fibroids, breast cysts, uterine cysts or tumors, endometriosis, pelvic organ prolapse (caused by a lack of muscular support for certain organs). Another issue can be constipation. Gonad Types tend to have cellulite, varicose veins, leg pain, and leg swelling and heaviness, including swollen ankles. They are also, often, overweight.

Gonad Types tend toward burnout as they neglect themselves by taking excessive care of others or working too hard.

They tend to have congestion along with a proper lack of circulation in their body — through their veins and sometimes in their lives.

Food Cravings: Beware of Nighttime Snacking

The Gonad Type has cravings after dinner and at night more often than at other times of the day. Cravings include:

- Mexican and/or other spicy food
- fatty or fried food
- butter, cream
- french fries, chips
- salty food
- red meat
- cold cuts
- red wine and other alcohol
- rosé or other creamy sauces and/or salad dressings
- peanut butter on toast

Cravings between 8 and 10 PM can be triggered by feelings of need, wanting affection, or the desire to have someone take care of them. Perhaps they feel their partner is not giving them enough attention. They'd do much better to ask for a hug rather than to indulge in food cravings.

Doing a detox is important to eliminate the toxins Gonad Types accumulate more easily than others. They also need to get their blood circulating by moving often. A mini trampoline may help to add movement breaks into a busy work day.

Strategy for the Gonad Type

Main Objective

Eating right for your body type will strengthen the pituitary and thyroid glands without causing an overstimulation of the ovaries that can hinder weight loss or cause abdominal bloating.

Reduce or eliminate all meals containing cream, butter, or any cooked fat. Protein must be eaten in moderation and mostly from chicken, fish, vegetarian protein and low-fat dairy products if these are tolerated by your body.

Low-fat yogurt and low-fat, low-sodium cottage cheese are excellent staples for the Gonad Type because they stimulate the pituitary gland.

One glass of skimmed milk at lunch time and again at dinner is good because it won't stimulate the gonads (ovaries) but will provide enough energy to eliminate hunger throughout the afternoon and evening. This is only recommended if you can digest milk products. If not, replace dairy with low-fat soy milk, almond milk, rice milk or another healthy milk alternative.

Eliminate Spicy, Stimulating Food

For the Gonad Type, black pepper, cayenne and other spices, such as hot peppers, are best avoided because they stimulate the ovaries. When we avoid overstimulating the dominant gland, the body is more balanced. As a result, we feel better, and weight loss happens more readily. Gonad Types can replace spices with aromatic herbs, such as thyme, sage, marjoram, tarragon, rosemary, parsley, fennel, and basil.

Eat Healthy Carbohydrates

Healthy carbohydrates stimulate the thyroid gland and allow the ovaries to rest. Consume a moderate amount of healthy carbohydrates from whole, unrefined grains or whole, stone-ground flours, such as buckwheat, millet, quinoa, spelt, Kamut Khorasan wheat, rye, brown rice, corn, or pasta made with whole-grain flours. Have a moderate amount of fruit as it also naturally stimulates the thyroid gland.

Eat Vegetables: Lots of Them!

Raw or cooked, enjoy vegetables in abundance.

Meals Best Suited to Gonad Type Energy

Breakfast Should Be Very Light

A little bit of fruit and herbal tea will do. If your breakfast is too large, you will build up an appetite and likely find yourself eating more than you should all day.

In one of the weight-loss groups I led, Cindy complained that her weight was staying the same. "That's because you're not following your body type's plan," I told her. She enjoyed bigger breakfasts with richer food, such as pâté with crackers. Like many Gonad Types, she was convinced there was no way she could last until lunch without a large breakfast. After weeks with no progress, she finally tried eating only a small piece of fruit for breakfast. The following week, Cindy shared how surprised she was that she wasn't hungry at all until lunch.

When explaining the Gonad Type plan to my clients, I tell them about breakfast **after** I've told them about all the great things they can eat at lunch and dinner because they are often upset to hear they do best with a small, light breakfast.

"But that's my favorite meal of the day," they exclaim. "You're not going to take away my peanut butter on toast, are you?"

Starting the day with a small, light breakfast will keep the Gonad Type feeling lighter and better all day long.

If you're having a breakfast smoothie, make sure it's not too thick: just fruit and skim milk, or an unsweetened milk alternative or even just a bit of water. Avoid adding nut butters, seeds, or any fat. Coffee is fine with skim milk or a milk alternative. Cream or even 2% milk is too heavy for you in the morning.

Light Lunch, Then Dinner Is the Main Meal

Lunch should also be light with a vegetarian protein, such as lentil or minestrone soup, or a bean salad. This will keep you feeling light but with the energy to stay productive throughout the afternoon.

Dinner is the main meal for the Gonad Type. Enjoy your favorite protein, either vegetarian protein or poultry or fish, good carbs such as potatoes, sweet potatoes or brown rice and lots of vegetables, cooked or raw. You can also add in a cup of unsweetened milk alternative and a few raw almonds if you like. Eating this way is most effective for weight loss and can help avoid late night snacking.

Portions: The Size of a Small Plate

Gonad Types need the least amount of food of any of the types. Small meals, about the size of a small plate, are key if you want to lose weight.

Alison found that everyone always remarked on how little she ate. When she tried to eat larger amounts, she often felt stuffed after dinner. I assured her that small portions were exactly what her Gonad Type needed. Once she cut down her servings, her digestion improved, she dropped 12 pounds, her joint pain disappeared, and she was able to sleep better.

The Gonad Type Plan: Light Breakfast, Early Supper

Breakfast: Around 8 AM

Options

- A small amount of fruit is the perfect breakfast for you. You may occasionally add a glass of skimmed milk, almond milk, or other milk alternative, or one of the options below.

- A small bowl of whole grain cereal with skim milk or a milk alternative. About a half a cup of cereal. In North America, Kamut Khorasan Wheat Flakes by Nature's Path is an excellent choice. A bowl of oatmeal is also good, but make sure to choose plain oats as the flavored variety can be high in sugar.
- A small (six-to-eight-ounce) smoothie made with various fruits, skim milk or unsweetened milk alternative or water. You can add greens or a protein powder occasionally. If you frequently work out, you may feel better with the protein powder at breakfast. Avoid adding nut butters or seeds as they are too heavy for you in the morning.

Lunch: Maximum of Four Hours Later

Optional Fruit

- a small portion (Fruit is more easily digested if eaten before vegetables.)

Vegetable Options

- a large salad (fresh vegetables and sprouts) with 1 tablespoon of homemade dressing containing extra virgin olive oil or vegetable oils that are cold-pressed
- a light, fat-free vegetable soup
- as many raw or cooked vegetables as you want

Protein Options

- a vegetarian meal with legumes such as lentils, chickpeas, kidney, or other beans, about ½ cup in all
- 2 oz of tofu
- 4 oz of fish
- 1 egg
- 1 cup of yogurt or 1 cup of low-fat cottage cheese (low-sodium)
- 4 oz of low-fat cheese, 7 percent fat or less, if none of the above options are available or you need an occasional change

Carbohydrate Options

- ½ cup of healthy carbohydrates (brown rice, quinoa, barley, millet, potatoes, pasta made from buckwheat, soy, spelt, Kamut Khorasan wheat, corn, or legumes)
- 1 slice of whole grain bread, preferably Kamut Khorasan wheat, spelt or rye

Optional Herbal Teas

- red clover or dandelion

Dinner: A Maximum of Five Hours after Lunch

As much as possible, dinner should be no later than 5 o'clock in the evening.

Optional Fruit

- A small fruit is optional while preparing dinner.

Vegetable Options

- a light, fat-free vegetable soup
- raw cooked vegetables (as much as you want) with 1 Tbsp of homemade dressing

Protein Options

- 4 oz of chicken or turkey
- 4 to 6 oz of fish
- 2 eggs
- Vegans or vegetarians can choose tempeh or tofu, which is high in protein, or lentils, chickpeas, kidney beans, or about ½ cup of other kinds of beans.

Carbohydrate Options

- ½ cup of healthy carbohydrates as above
- a slice of whole-grain or Kamut Khorasan wheat bread

Optional Herbal Teas

- red clover or dandelion

Other Suggestions for The Gonad Type

The Importance of an Early Dinner

Most Gonad Type clients tell me that as soon as they get home from work around 5 o'clock, they want to eat everything in sight. They might nibble on crackers and cheese *and* sample dinner as they make it. Some eat so much that they're no longer hungry at mealtime. Other types may be able to eat later, but not you. Five o'clock is the perfect dinnertime because that's when you are ready for a full meal. If you find it impossible to eat that early, try to do so as early as possible (even if that means eating ahead of others) because that will make you feel best and make it easiest to drop unwanted pounds.

If you work late, have a snack mid-afternoon so you're not overly hungry at dinner. Eat dinner earlier on the nights you don't work.

Get Your Sleep and Learn to Say 'No'

It is worth re-emphasizing that the Gonad Type needs more sleep than any of the other types. Tuck yourself into bed early and sleep in late on weekends if possible. As I noted earlier, the Gonad Type is the motherly, caregiving, generous type. That will never change! However, you also need to carve out some time to take care of yourself. Learn to give *and* receive; don't overbook yourself, allocate time for your own needs, and learn to say no. Remember the sage advice given to mothers by airline flight attendants: put on your own oxygen mask before helping others with theirs. Don't wait until a health scare shakes you up to start changing your ways.

Sylvie, a Gonad Type mom with two teenaged boys, found herself in the hospital before she started her journey of self-care. Fortunately, her problem wasn't too serious, and she was able to join one of my weight loss groups.

A busy attorney who commuted by train, she began to plan and prepare a lot of the week's dinners on the weekends. She also went to the gym two to three times a week. By following her body type's plan, she dropped 15 pounds in 12 weeks. "Who are you and what have you done with my wife?" her husband asked her.

If I had a magic wand, all Gonad Types would spend as much time taking care of themselves as they do others. When we transform our health and lives for the better, it makes everyone around us happier.

Work Your Upper Body and Get Your Blood Flowing

Exercise that involves strengthening the upper body and improving blood circulation is best. Activities may include:

- aerobics
- dancing
- t'ai chi
- badminton
- volleyball
- yoga
- mini-trampoline workouts to help the lymphatic system (This is recommended only for those with strong pelvic floor muscles.)

It is best to avoid exercises that focus on the lower body, such as skating, jogging, cycling, and mountain climbing. While any kind of exercise is better than none, Gonad Types who do something like spinning classes often could end up bulking up their lower body. Choosing exercises that strengthen the upper body will help drop unwanted pounds more easily.

Vitamins and Supplements

It's hard to get everything we need from our diet. Vitamins and supplements can help cover your nutritional bases, keep your bones strong, promote healthy aging, reduce anxiety and stress, boost your health, and more. Before you start any vitamin or supplement, **always** check with your physician and/or pharmacist to make sure that none of these supplements will worsen any pre-existing conditions or counteract with any of your existing medications.

- Red Raspberry tonic may help regulate the female organs.
- Ginger, a warming root, is known to help improve circulation, which is beneficial because the Gonad Type can be prone to congestion. It may also be good for digestive disturbances and, as a natural anti-spasmodic, it may help with menstrual cramps, hormonal headaches, and hormonal acne.
- Siberian Ginseng can stimulate the adrenal glands and help with stress. Take as prescribed for one month at a time, and then take a break for one month, then repeat.
- Butcher's broom is known to clean and tone veins, as the Gonad Type tends toward varicose veins.
- Ginkgo biloba is known to enhance circulation.
- Potassium is good for the heart.
- Dandelion may help purify the blood; it's also good for arthritis and liver function.
- Plant-based digestive enzymes can help break down food and improve digestion.
- Supplements, such as kelp that is high in iodine, can support the thyroid gland.

Herbal Tea Suggestions

Red clover tea is traditionally used to balance hormones, making it a perfect choice for Gonad Types. Dandelion, a bitter herb that has cleansing and nourishing properties, is known to help digestion, improve liver function, and remove toxins from the muscles, joints, and weak areas in the body.

Adrenal Type

Adrenal Type: The Sociable One

I love working with Adrenal Types. Lively go-getters, they are fun to be around, and there is no stopping an Adrenal Type when they have harnessed their determination. Some struggle with being overweight because they *love* food! This can make portion control difficult.

Marie-Claude was an Adrenal Type in my weight loss group, who ate overly large portions. When I paired up the participants for buddy support, Marie-Claude often texted her buddy, exclaiming, "I'm hungry! I'm hungry!" Her buddy was not sure how to respond but encouraged her to keep to her Bodytypology plan.

After two weeks, Marie-Claude's body adjusted, and she didn't feel as hungry. "I noticed I wasn't craving salt as much anymore," she noted. "And now that I've completed the program, I don't overeat — even when it's delicious — because I have no longer have any interest in getting that overstuffed feeling." Following her body type's plan, Marie-Claude lost fifteen pounds by the end of the twelve-week session.

The Adrenal Type is the strongest of the four types and they enjoy using their strength. An Adrenal Type easily rearranges the furniture or refuses help when carrying heavy bags of groceries. Some are reserved and quiet, although they hold their ground when necessary.

Energy Levels are Stable

Adrenal Types have large energy reserves, but they're not typically morning people. They likely prefer to stay in bed longer when given the opportunity, such as on weekends, to quietly enjoy their coffee without being disturbed. Although they can be slow in the morning, particularly if they've stayed up too late or eaten a large meal or snack just before bedtime, they are ready to put the show on the road if need be.

An Adrenal Type's energy is generally stable all day and they tend to have more energy at night. They may stay up until 11 or midnight regularly without it affecting their overall energy level.

Overall, an Adrenal Type body is like a diesel truck: hard to start up, but once going, it's hard to stop. While other types might end up exhausted, even burned out, from a hardship or extreme stress, the sturdy Adrenal Type keeps on trucking.

Personality Traits: Calm on the Outside, Nervous Inside

The Adrenal Type is warm, jovial, and sociable — the life of the party! They help everyone out and are appreciated by many. They tend to enjoy team sports.

Although Adrenal Types seem to handle stress well, underneath that calm, cool exterior there is a gnawing, nervous energy. This needs to be addressed for weight loss to be successful. Our bodies hold on to the extra weight for protection unless we learn to better manage stress.

This book's section on stress management offers some quieter and, perhaps, healthier strategies.

Adrenal Types may not be as creative as Thyroid Types, but they believe they can succeed at most anything. Practical and down to earth, Adrenal Type people are able to be objective most times and have a high level of tolerance for other people and difficult situations.

Stability is the strength of the Adrenal Type person so they like everyone and everything else to be stable as well. They generally don't like unpredictable or impromptu events and they don't appreciate changes in their schedule. That said, they also don't like to be restricted by too many 'musts' or 'shoulds'.

An Adrenal Type reading this passage may well be impatient with all this personality description because they don't like to analyze themselves or others. Abstractions that require creativity, imagination and/or reflection are not their favorite pastimes.

Although Adrenal Types excel at being stable and hardworking; they tend to burn the candle at both ends. They want to come out the winner in all situations, discussions, competitions, and even arguments. As a result, they can be overly sure of themselves and tend to give quick short answers rather than having the patience for longer explanations, even when more detail is needed.

Beware of the Adrenal Type anger as they can become rigid, inflexible and stubborn — even to the point of being dominating or authoritarian. They tend to have major blow-ups when annoyed.

The gland of anger is the liver, and this kind of temperament can show up and be exacerbated when the liver is overworked from consuming too much red meat, fatty food, and/or alcohol.

These emotions tend to make Adrenal Types react quickly. When they are hungry, it is best not to talk to them until after they have eaten.

It's beneficial for Adrenal Types to learn to stop pushing themselves and instead recognize and accept their vulnerabilities.

Physical Traits: Solid, Strong, and Large Chested

An Adrenal Type is big-boned, stocky, solid, strong and, in some cases, short. Their upper body is dominant. Adrenal men are built like football players while Adrenal women tend to have a large chest (think of Oprah Winfrey). Adrenal Type women tend to have breasts that are round like apples, rather than pear-shaped. Their waist and thighs are not easily distinguished from each other. When physically fit, Adrenal Types have muscular arms and legs, a straight back, and small buttocks. Sometimes their legs can be quite thin compared to their upper body. When they gain weight, it tends to be more in the upper body, chest, abdomen — especially the upper abdomen right under the chest rather than the lower belly. However, gravity may cause some to have a belly that sags. They also tend to accumulate fat on their back.

An Adrenal Type's muscle mass increases easily. They tend to enjoy sports that build their arms and upper body, such as lifting heavy weights or paddle-boarding. They have a high metabolism and radiate a lot of body heat. They also often blush and become red-faced when angry, overly heated, or when they exert themselves. Some Adrenal Types also tend to have oily skin and a young appearance.

Adrenal Types are known to have a high tolerance for physical pain.

Common Ailments: Cholesterol and Cardiovascular Issues

The weak points on an Adrenal-Type body are the liver and the heart. Those who have a high fat diet and neglect their health, can run into problems with their cardiovascular system — high blood pressure, heart attacks, strokes, high cholesterol, and blocked arteries. Also, their gall bladders may be prone to stones. And finally, an Adrenal-Type person with a weak thyroid gland will tend to be depressed.

Many of these conditions tend to go undetected and are known as silent killers. It's important to check cardiovascular health and thyroid levels with a doctor.

With a tendency toward excess, Adrenal Types are also susceptible to liver congestion. When the liver is congested, fatigue and poor digestion can set in. Adrenal Types need to be careful of excessive lifestyle choices that can lead to diabetes, alcoholism, gout, and overall exhaustion.

Food Cravings: Salt and Fat

Many Adrenal Types favor salty food over sweets, although some go for both. In excess, salty food can create bloating. If an Adrenal-Type person craves sweets, it might be rich pastries, creamy dishes, sugar pie, caramel sauce, and the like. They tend to like red meat, fatty food, and alcohol, especially red wine. Eating and drinking tend to give them a feeling of strength, so they need to be careful not to overindulge.

Norman was an Adrenal Type who was following his plan and was dropping a pound or two each week. One week he visited my office excited to share that he had read the information I had provided on emotional eating and realized that he was emotional drinking. Since his father's passing a few years earlier, he had been using alcohol to numb his sadness.

"I got so much more out of this experience than I expected," he says. "I now understand the *why* behind some of my bad habits."

My primary goal for my clients is to uncover the underlying cause of any weight gain and release the usually associated pain with it for their long-term success. (More about this later.)

The Adrenal Type leans towards excess of all kinds, and these can include:

- chips and other salty food
- pastries, chocolate, and other sweets
- fatty food
- fried food
- popcorn
- fried eggs
- rich sauces
- peanuts
- cheese
- cold cuts
- toast with butter, never plain
- red meat, including the fat
- alcohol, especially red wine
- food marinated in vinegar with salt

Adrenal Types tend to want to eat fatty, salty, or cheesy food around 4 PM and at night when their energy is waning. They rarely drink enough water or eat sufficient fruit and vegetables.

Strategy for the Adrenal Type

Main Objective

By eating right for your body type, you'll strengthen the pituitary and thyroid glands while allowing your adrenals to rest. To do this, it is necessary to eliminate red meat as much as possible. Choose poultry, fish, or non-meat sources of protein, such as beans, lentils, chickpeas, or kidney beans instead.

If you want to lose weight, reduce or eliminate salt and fat. (Yes, we do need *some* salt. Sun dried sea salt from France is a good choice.)

Reduce cold cuts, marinades and creamy sauces. In eating right for your body type, you are strengthening your weaker glands, such as the pituitary and thyroid, while not overworking the adrenals.

Ensure that all meals are as free of fat as possible. For instance, cut any excess fat off meat, don't eat the skin on chicken, and reduce butter and sauce intake. Keeping your intake of healthy fats, such as nuts, seeds, and avocados, to a minimum is also important to help your body drop those excess pounds.

I know there are some Adrenal Types reading this and thinking I just took away your favorite kinds of food. In a way, that's true. Each of the four body types craves foods that stimulate their dominant gland, which causes the body to be unbalanced. The truth is we often crave what is not good for us because we often interpret our cravings incorrectly. We might think we need sugar for a boost when we are tired, but we really need protein. However, when you start following your body type's plan, your cravings will diminish.

When clients are struggling with cravings, I usually suggest that they have two deviations per week. (I never use the word 'cheat' as it has such a negative connotation.)

It will get easier, I promise.

The amount of weight you lose will coincide with how closely you adhere to your body type's plan. If you are maintaining your ideal weight, you will still reap all the benefits by feeling more balanced, energetic, and having an overall feeling of well-being, along with reduced cravings.

Eat Good Quality Carbohydrates

Good quality carbohydrates stimulate the thyroid gland and allow the adrenals to rest. Cereals and whole grain products should be made with unrefined, unbleached flour that is preferably stone-ground to retain its nutritional benefits. A good choice is Nature's Path Kamut Khorasan Wheat Flakes. With only five grams of sugar, this cereal keeps all my Adrenal-Type clients satisfied until lunch. Choose whole grain brown rice, rye, buckwheat, corn, quinoa, spelt, Kamut Khorasan wheat, barley, or millet rather than wheat or oats.

Eat various legumes, such as black beans, lentils, chickpeas, as well as potatoes and sweet potatoes, or pasta made from whole grains.

Have Some Low–Fat Dairy if You Can Tolerate It

For many people, dairy is not recommended as it increases mucus production. This is the body's natural way to protect itself when it doesn't tolerate a particular food or other substance. You might find your nose dripping often or have extra mucus at the back of your throat.

One of my clients had a chronic cough for 10 years, something that she said the many different types of doctors she visited weren't able to resolve. Suspecting there was a substance irritating her body, I suggested she give up wheat and dairy for a few weeks. She was ecstatic when, soon after, her excess mucus stopped and her cough disappeared. Her husband was also grateful to not have to listen to her coughing!

Adrenal Types who do tolerate dairy can have limited amounts of skim milk, low fat or Greek yogurt, as well as low fat or ricotta cheese, as these stimulate the thyroid and pituitary glands. Low-fat cottage cheese is high in protein, but it's also high in sodium. Low-sodium cottage cheese may be hard to find. Frozen yogurt once or twice a week may be a good treat, but make sure the sugar content isn't too high.

If you do not tolerate dairy well, unsweetened almond milk, rice milk, coconut milk, or soy milk can be good alternatives. Avoid oat milk as it is usually thickened with refined oil.

Eat Plenty of Vegetables

As they say, "Eat the colors of the rainbow," raw or cooked, in abundance. About five servings or more per day. About ½ cup cooked or 1 cup raw per serving.

Drink Lots of Water

It is often challenging for the Adrenal Type to drink enough water. I am constantly reminding my partner to drink more water; he just doesn't think of it.

As the saying goes, "Water is the solution for the dilution of the pollution", so make every effort to increase water consumption. Start with a minimum of 4 cups per day and gradually increase to about half your body weight in ounces.

Meals Best Suited to Adrenal Type Energy

The size and quality of your meals should follow your metabolism level, which increases as the day progresses.

A Light Breakfast

A smoothie or whole grain cereal with milk (skim or low fat, unsweetened soy milk, almond milk, or rice milk).

When you consume a heavy breakfast such as bacon and eggs or partake in a big breakfast buffet, the adrenal glands that are inactive in the morning will become overstimulated, triggering you to feel hungry and sluggish for the rest of the day.

Lunch Is Also Light

A salad or vegetables with a good quality carbohydrate and fruit. A vegetarian lunch, with a protein such as lentils, quinoa, chickpeas or other beans, is perfect for Adrenal Type energy and will keep you more balanced throughout the afternoon. If you must have animal protein, choose fish, and avoid the energy slump you would have if you ate a lunch with red meat.

Dinner Is the Main Meal

This is the time of day that Adrenal Types can best handle a full meal. Your metabolism is highest, so the meal will burn off more easily. This simply means you can better digest a more substantial protein, such as chicken. The portion size should not be larger than a normal plate. By making dinner the main meal of the day, your appetite is more easily controlled. You can get into the habit of giving your body lighter, smaller meals when you tend to be less hungry, and larger meals when you're hungrier. Adrenal Types who do this will find that their energy remains stable and well balanced throughout the day.

Avoid snacking late at night if your goal is weight loss. Late night snacks add calories you don't need.

The Adrenal Type Plan

Breakfast: Around 8 AM

Options

- A small bowl (½ to 1 cup) of whole grain cereal with skim milk or a milk alternative. In North America, Kamut Khorasan Wheat Flakes by Nature's Path is an excellent choice. A bowl of oatmeal is also good, but make sure to choose plain oats, as the flavored variety can be high in sugar
- 1 cup of low fat or Greek yogurt with 1/2 cup of whole grain cereal
- 1 oz of low-fat cheese with a slice of whole-grain bread, preferably made with Kamut Khorasan wheat, spelt, or rye flour
- a smoothie made with about a cup of various fruits, skim milk or a milk alternative or water (You also can add leafy greens or a protein powder.)

- herbal tea suggestions: chamomile or parsley

Avoid fried food or nut butters as they are too heavy for you to digest in the morning.

Lunch: Maximum of Four Hours Later

Optional Fruit
A small fruit (Remember that fruit is more easily digested if eaten before your meal.)

Vegetable Options

- a large salad (fresh vegetables and sprouts) with 1 Tbsp homemade dressing containing extra virgin olive oil or oils that are cold-pressed
- a light, fat-free vegetable soup
- as many raw and/or cooked vegetables as you want

Protein Options

- 5 oz of fish
- a vegetarian meal with ½ cup of legumes such as lentils, chickpeas, kidney beans or other kinds of beans
- 1 cup of yogurt
- 1 cup of cottage cheese (low-sodium, if possible)
- 1 egg
- if none of these choices are available, 4 oz of low-fat cheese, 7% fat or less

Carbohydrate Options

- ½ cup good quality carbohydrates (brown rice, quinoa, barley, millet, potatoes, beans, pasta made from buckwheat, soy, spelt, Kamut Khorasan wheat, corn or legumes)
- one slice of whole grain bread, preferably Kamut Khorasan wheat, spelt or rye

Optional Herbal Teas

- chamomile or parsley

Dinner: Maximum Six Hours After Lunch

Dinner should be no later than six o'clock in the evening.

Optional Fruit

- If you are preparing dinner and feel hungry, this would be the perfect time to have a small serving of fruit.

Vegetable Options

- a light fat-free, vegetable soup
- raw and/or cooked vegetables (as much as you want) with 1 Tbsp of homemade dressing containing extra virgin olive oil or vegetable oils that are cold-pressed

Protein Options

- 4 oz of chicken or turkey
- 6 oz of fish
- 2 eggs
- Vegans or vegetarians can choose 6 oz of tempeh or tofu, which is high in protein, or lentils, chickpeas, kidney beans, or other kinds of beans.

Carbohydrate Options

- ½ cup of good quality carbohydrates (see pg 50)
- a slice of whole-grain or Kamut Khorasan wheat bread

Optional Herbal Teas

- chamomile or parsley

Other Suggestions for the Adrenal Type

Don't Be Shy About Getting Help to Handle Stress

Adrenal Types tend to internalize stress. When the body is under a lot of stress, it will hold on to fat to protect itself.

One of my clients managed a post office and felt a huge amount of stress to serve her customers as quickly as possible all day long. Her husband remarked that even when she was at home, she was like a ping pong ball, bouncing around the house from project to project, always in a tizzy. Even though she followed her plan, she lost very little weight. Her body held the fat to deal with her constant state of high stress. She worked hard at changing her eating patterns and exercising, but ultimately, the weight never did come off, leaving her frustrated and saying to herself, "my body just won't drop the weight."

Working with a therapist could be beneficial to determine and release the underlying causes of continued high levels of stress.

Watch Those Portions

Pay attention to portion control, which is often a challenge for Adrenal Types. Serve yourself a regular portion and put away the food before sitting down to eat to check that tendency of going back for seconds. Serve snacks in a small bowl or a plate instead of eating from the package.

Get Your Sleep

Get enough sleep. Some Adrenal types are able to stay up and tend to burn the candle at both ends, resulting in being sleep deprived. Lack of sleep has been proven to hinder weight loss. Some theories suggest lack of sleep can lead to impulsive behaviour, such as late-night snacking.

Give Your Liver Some Love

Take care of your liver by avoiding chemicals, additives, poor-quality fat (found in processed foods and deep-fried foods), excess alcohol, and unnecessary medication. A 30-day detox is very beneficial for Adrenal Types because you often have a congested liver. (See the detox section p. 23.)

Let's Say it Again! Have a Glass (or 8!) of Water

Drink plenty of water — a real challenge. Most Adrenal-Type people I've helped simply don't think of drinking water. You need constant reminders. Drinking hot water with the juice of half a lemon first thing in the morning is excellent to help the liver detox.

Remember: the goal is to develop a lifelong water-drinking habit, so start with a realistic amount, about 4 glasses, and then add to it gradually.

Work on Your Flexibility and Speed

In general, Adrenal types have a strong upper body. However, your body tends to get stiff. Any sport or exercise that requires flexibility and/or speed to get you moving is best for you. These activities include:

- tennis
- badminton
- squash
- ping pong
- yoga

It is best to avoid excessive workouts aimed at increasing upper body muscle mass, as that part of your body is generally already.

Vitamins and Supplements

Most people don't get the seven to ten organic fruits and vegetables needed every day for a balanced diet, so taking vitamins and supplements can be beneficial. Before you start any vitamin or supplement, **always** check with your physician and/or pharmacist to make sure that none of these supplements will worsen any pre-existing conditions or counteract with any of your existing medications.

- Complex B: calms the nervous system
- Vitamin C: supports the adrenal glands
- Digestive enzymes: to help break down food (Insufficient enzymes can result in bloating, gas, or constipation.)
- Depending on the individual, herbs that help to cleanse the liver (see the detox section p. 23)
- Potassium: good for the heart and may help prevent hypertension

Herbal Tea Suggestions

Chamomile tea is calming. Parsley has a refreshing astringent quality and may satisfy your desire for a savory taste. Use 2 tsp of dried or 2 Tbsp fresh parsley per cup of tea. Steep in boiled water for 5 minutes then strain. You can add lemon and/or a touch of honey if you wish.

Thyroid Type

Thyroid Type: Beware of the Roller Coaster

Vivacious, quick learners and entrepreneurial, Thyroid Types generally have a roller coaster kind of energy throughout the day, which can have a real impact on their mood. You are likely a Thyroid Type if you are tall and thin with long arms and legs. If you gain weight, it tends to be around the middle of your body.

Energy Levels: Watch Out for the 4PM Slump

As I mentioned at the start of the book, the Thyroid Type was the first body type presented in my naturopathy classes, and I was amazed at how accurately it described me at that time. My energy constantly went up and down. I was tired before and sometimes after lunch and especially around four o'clock. I was always hungry and snacking a lot. I was struggling with low blood-sugar levels given how irritable I would get whenever I would go without eating for too long.

For 16 years, I had been vegetarian (similar to many Thyroid Types). As a yoga instructor, I stubbornly refused to eat animal protein. It went against everything I believed.

My naturopathy teacher said I wasn't getting enough protein for my body type. I learned that protein stimulates the adrenal glands that give us energy. After many weeks of learning about the benefits of eating right for our body type, I decided to give poultry a try. Then I started integrating fish and more eggs into my meals. My energy and strength both gradually increased. My afternoon slumps disappeared.

For us Thyroid Types, it's early to bed, early to rise. Morning is the best time of the day. We wake up early, often six o'clock or six-thirty without an alarm clock, ready to take on the world! However, I, for one, can't start any new projects after 9 pm as my focus and energy wane.

You may think you're a morning person because you're up and at 'em at 6 AM making breakfast and getting the kids and yourself ready for the day, but that may be out of necessity rather than choice. The real question is: How late do you sleep on weekends if no one wakes you up? For a Thyroid Type, this would be seven or eight o'clock at the latest.

With real highs and then lows in terms of energy, Thyroid Types often rely on stimulants, such as coffee, tea, cigarettes, chocolate, other sweets, or carbs to re-boost themselves. Their cravings become strongest when their energy is low. They typically have an energy crash around 4 or 4:30 PM. Their energy can also be low mid-morning (around 10:30 AM). Then their energy may increase after dinner, but drop back down at bedtime. If they are hypoglycemic (low blood-sugar level), they may wake, possibly from a nightmare, around 4 AM. This is often the case for children who enjoy too many sweets without enough protein for dinner. Some Thyroid Types, who tend to have a light dinner lacking in protein, may also have trouble falling asleep and then remaining in a sound sleep.

Most Thyroid Types do not fare well with staying up late. They are ready for bed by 10 or 10:30 PM. If they do have a late night, they will feel tired most of the next day, and it can take a couple of days of proper rest to recuperate.

Personality Traits: A Passion for Novelty

The thyroid gland is the gland of feelings, sentimentality, movement, and rapidity. If you are feeling depressed, or sad, or preoccupied by fearful thoughts, it could be an indication that your thyroid is unbalanced.

Decorum is very important to Thyroid Types, who tend to judge people and things by appearance. Keeping things in order keeps them more at ease.

The Thyroid is also the gland of adaptability, vitality, and delicacy. This type thrives on change. They love starting new projects or hobbies and have a passion for new adventures and will likely enjoy traveling to somewhere new rather than returning to the same place each year. In their enthusiasm for new things, they tend to leave projects unfinished as they move onto their next venture.

Thyroid Types express themselves well and many are writers. They may use their hands to gesture a lot as they talk.

They take sentimental letdowns, heartbreaks, divorce, and other types of division harder than most people. Being rejected is a Thyroid Type's Achilles' heel. It is interesting to note that most people — regardless of type — experience the loss of a loved one, or a significant job, right before being diagnosed with hypothyroidism, which indicates the strong correlation between emotional strife and the thyroid gland's imbalance.

Thyroid Types hate dealing with seemingly insurmountable problems; regular sources of frustration; the feeling of overwhelm; the need for too much thinking; any boring routines or monotony; as well as situations requiring power, stability, and endurance. They can feel as if they lack stability because they have difficulty seeing things long-term, which leaves them feeling insecure. They tend to work too hard because it is hard for them to be idle, although they are easily distracted. When pregnant, they tend to feel trapped and can't wait to start doing their own thing again.

Thyroid Types are also easily drawn into excess, and they don't tend to eat a healthy diet.

While highly sensitive, Thyroid Types can be insensitive toward others. Their moods change quickly, from pumped up with excitement to feeling down, even defeated; from whirlwind and creative to negative and destructive. They often have a nervous energy, may talk a lot and quickly, and they may tend to exaggerate.

When angry, their fury is most often directed at the situation rather than a person. Nevertheless, they tend to be abrupt and get straight to the point of most everything, which not everyone appreciates. It is not a good idea to contradict Thyroid Type people because their memory is strong.

The most mercurial traits of Thyroid Types come out when they are low on energy. They are much more likely to be diplomatic when they're enjoying a healthy balance. To do this, they need to get outside a lot to enjoy fresh air, learn to rest, and go on vacations more often.

Physical Traits: Delicate Bones and Dry Skin

Thyroid Types have a delicate appearance, with thin bones, a small face, and narrow neck. They tend to have dry skin and their hair is also dry and breaks easily. They tend to go grey earlier than others — generally around age 40 or sooner.

If they have any excess weight, it generally accumulates around the middle, on the stomach and/or lower abdomen. They tend to have soft low abdomen fat — what we often call a spare tire — around the middle with curves and rolls of flesh. They also gain weight on their hips and upper thighs and don't tend to gain in the face, arms, or legs. Their lower back is straight, and buttocks are round but not pronounced. Thyroid Type women do not develop cellulite, which is a key way to determine their type. Also, they perspire very little.

Common Ailments: Watch the Blood Sugar!

Thyroid types are prone to hypoglycemia, diabetes, and ailments involving the nervous system, such as headaches or dizziness, as well as digestive issues. The digestive system is directly related to the nervous system and many digestive ailments originate from emotional issues, stress and/or anxiety.

Because they take on too much, they use stimulants and sweets to keep going, which can lead to burnout, depression, colitis, ulcers, cramps, intestinal spasms, diarrhea or constipation. They are prone to poor digestion, heart burn, as well as acid reflux. Their body is often overly acidic. To buffer the acidity, the body may leach calcium from the bones, magnesium from the nerves, potassium from the muscles, and sodium from the joints and digestive tract, leaving the body in a weakened, disease-prone state. This leaves an unbalanced Thyroid Type prone to osteoporosis and joint pain or skin problems such as eczema.

When I was studying to be a naturopath, I learned how to check my pH level by testing my saliva and urine over five days. My acidity levels were off the charts! I learned how to reduce the acidity by increasing my consumption of alkalinizing food, such as dark leafy greens. I also worked at managing my stress better and started dry-brushing my skin to exfoliate it, unclog the pores, and detoxify. I started taking aloe vera juice and chlorophyll supplements.

The eczema I had on my hands for 20 years disappeared, never to return. My ghostly complexion also began to take on a healthy glow. Every time I looked in the mirror, I was surprised to see such rosy cheeks.

The Thyroid Type is prone to fears: fear of emptiness, insecurity, claustrophobia, nervous tics. They rarely have high blood pressure, although they may have palpitations or tachycardia. They are also sensitive to touch. For example, they can be very sensitive about having dental work done.

It is also common to suffer from fatigue. Thyroid Type people need to recuperate, reset and recharge on a regular basis.

Food Cravings: Sweets and Stimulants

Sweets and stimulants are a Thyroid Type's downfall. They often crave some of the following:

- coffee
- sugar
- chocolate
- fruit
- alcohol, particularly wine
- caffeinated tea
- cigarettes
- carbohydrates, bread, pasta, starches
- soda / pop drinks

Cravings tend to be strongest at 10:30 AM, 4:30 PM and before bedtime.

They have a good, large appetite and generally a fast digestive system and are fortunate in that they do not tend to gain weight as much as some of the other types.

Strategy for the Thyroid Type

Main Objective

Eating right for your body type will strengthen the adrenal glands and gonads (ovaries or testicles) without overstimulating the thyroid. Possible symptoms of an overactive thyroid include nervousness, anxiety, irritability, and mood swings. You may find it hard to stay still and have a lot of nervous energy. All body types gravitate towards foods that stimulate your dominant gland whenever you feel tired, pressured, or stressed, but Thyroid Types are particularly vulnerable to this tendency. The Thyroid Type already tends to have a lot of nervous energy and adding stimulants to the mix exacerbates this problem. Follow your body type's plan and you can look forward to calmer, more even energy throughout the day.

Eliminate Refined Carbohydrates and Sweets

Not all carbs are equal. For example, white rice is brown rice that has been milled and polished, removing the outer layer that contains all the nutrients in the bran, germ, and endo sperm. Brown rice is higher in protein, fiber, fats, and vitamins and minerals. It's time to shift your focus to healthy carbohydrates, such as brown rice, quinoa, and sweet potatoes, in moderate amounts. One serving equals about a ½ cup.

Reduce and eliminate

- sweets (including candies);
- chocolate;
- pastries, cakes, and other desserts;

- soda / pop drinks;
- any other sugary drinks;
- fruit juices;
- white rice;
- white flour; and
- white sugar and anything containing it.

Sweets and refined carbs stimulate the thyroid gland, giving you the exhilarating fix that you crave by spiking up your energy. However, they also send you on a roller coaster of blood sugar ups and downs all day long. When your blood sugar has these peaks and valleys, so do your moods. I know this personally. By eliminating or at least cutting back on refined sweets and increasing your protein intake, you will feel so much more balanced.

If your goal is to lose weight, eliminate all bread while on this plan until your desired weight is reached. Then reintroduce bread in small quantities, preferably Kamut Khorasan or spelt sourdough. When you eat healthy carbohydrates, have about half a cup from whole unrefined grains or whole stone-ground flours, such as buckwheat, millet, quinoa, spelt, Kamut Khorasan wheat, rye, brown rice, corn, or pasta made with whole-grain flours.

Eliminate Wheat and Oats

For you, wheat and oats are more quickly transformed into fat while complete cereals (brown rice, corn, quinoa, millet, spelt, Kamut Khorasan wheat, rye, and buckwheat) help you to build muscle instead.

Avoid Fruit During This Plan

Avoiding fruit may seem odd since fruit is generally considered healthy for us, but for the Thyroid Type, fruit contains too much simple sugar that stimulates the thyroid gland. Eliminating or at least significantly reducing your fruit intake will help to curb your cravings for sweets.

Meals Best Suited to Thyroid Type Energy

Three Full Meals a Day

Each meal should contain a complete protein to maintain stable energy all day long. Never skip or delay a meal. This is important, especially with breakfast. Making sure that you always have breakfast will change your life. It did mine...

My mom made us five kids a full breakfast with cereal, toast, and a different kind of egg every day when we were young. We never needed to eat anything at recess like the other kids did. In high school, I started eating only cereal because it was fast and easy. I'd be so hungry by mid-morning that I'd eat the two sandwiches I had packed for lunch and then go to a friend's house and eat two more sandwiches at noon.

When I waitressed at a French bistro in my twenties, I was always reaching for bread or snacking on something else.

"Stop eating!" the maître d' warned. "You're going to gain weight."

After I had been working there for several weeks, he marveled that I was *always eating* but never gained weight. My nervous energy and fast metabolism burned all the food off, but I was always hungry and often irritable and anxious.

You may have tall, slim friends who can eat all they want and never gain weight. Don't you just hate that? No doubt they're a Thyroid Type. If you're a Thyroid Type, you may be blessed with a fast metabolism, but you're not immune to gaining weight, especially if you succumb to your sweet and carb cravings. I eat healthily, sticking to my Thyroid Type plan, and I do plenty of outdoor exercise to maintain my ideal weight.

When I started eating right for my Thyroid Type, including two eggs for breakfast every day, I felt so much more balanced, calm, and satisfied food-wise all day.

The Thyroid Type Plan

Breakfast: Around 8 AM

Eating eggs daily is highly recommended for the Thyroid Type. This will help you start off with adequate protein and leave you feeling satisfied throughout the day. If you are concerned about cholesterol, keeping the yolk runny leads to a negligible effect on cholesterol levels.

Options

- 2 eggs with runny yolks (poached or soft boiled)
- 4 oz of chicken
- 4 oz of homemade pâté or cretons from chicken, turkey, or veal
- vegans or vegetarians: 4 oz of veggie pâté, tofu scramble, or a vegetarian protein such as a bean burrito
- vegetables, if desired
- herbal tea: raspberry leaf or rosehips

A Snack if Needed Around 10 or 10:30 AM

- nuts
- organic yogurt or kefir
- a home-made power bar (See recipe section p.129)

Lunch: A Maximum of Four Hours After Breakfast

Vegetable Options

- a large salad (fresh vegetables, sprouts) with 1 Tbsp homemade dressing made with extra virgin olive oil or vegetable oils that are first pressed cold

- a light, fat-free vegetable soup
- as many raw or cooked vegetables as you want

Protein Options

- 4 oz of a complete protein, such as chicken, fish, or an organic red meat
- Vegans or vegetarians can choose 4 oz of tempeh or tofu, which is high in protein, or ½ cup of lentils, chickpeas, kidney beans or other legumes.

Carbohydrate Options

- ½ cup healthy carbohydrates, such as brown rice, millet, potatoes, barley, beans, pasta made from buckwheat, soya, spelt, Kamut Khorasan wheat, corn or legumes.

Optional Extras

- ½ cup of yogurt, or
- 1 cup of skim milk, if your system tolerates dairy well

Optional Herbal Teas

- raspberry leaf or rosehip herbal tea

Must-Have Protein Snack Around 4 PM
(Be Sure to Have It Before Your Energy Crashes!)

- ½ cup plain yogurt
- a large handful of trail mix with organic raw ingredients (See Recipe section p. 136)
- about 1/3 cup hummus with any veggies
- 1 homemade power bar (See recipe section p.129)

Dinner: A Maximum of Six Hours After Lunch

Vegetable Options

- a light, fat-free vegetable soup or as many raw and/or cooked vegetables as you want

Protein Options

- 4 oz of a complete protein, such as chicken, fish, or an organic red meat
- Vegans or vegetarians can choose 4 oz of tempeh or tofu, which is high in protein, or lentils, chickpeas, kidney beans, or other kinds of beans.

Carbohydrate Options

- ½ cup carbohydrates (see pg 64)

Optional extras

- ½ cup of yogurt or 1 cup of skim milk if your system tolerates dairy well

Optional Herbal Teas

- raspberry leaf or rosehip herbal tea

Other Suggestions for the Thyroid Type

Rest Rather than Stimulants

Once you have reached your weight goal (if that was your initial goal for eating for your body type), an occasional coffee or some fruit is fine, but you need to stop relying on these stimulants for energy and instead get more rest. Staying away from sugar is essential as it's like a drug for Thyroid Types. That is certainly the case for me. I don't keep any sweets in the house. I ask my boyfriend to hide his dark chocolate. I rarely bake unless it's for someone's get-together or we're having guests.

Jennifer was a Thyroid Type who began every day with a 10 o'clock breakfast of wheat toast and lots of jam. Bagels with cream cheese were a favorite late lunch, along with cookies for snacks. A week after implementing her plan, including the eggs for breakfast, she said she felt much better: less bloated and gassy, less moody, and she had a lot more energy.

You'll feel much better if you tuck in early. If you do stay up late, it usually takes a day or two to recuperate.

Sit and Stand Tall!

Also sit and stand tall! Long and lanky Thyroid Types have a tendency to slouch. It is so important to pull back your shoulders and sit up straight so that you maintain a strong upright stance to avoid posture and balance issues as you get older.

No Need for Speed, Overall Strength Instead

General training is best to develop strength and increase muscle mass. Ideal activities include the following:

- swimming
- rowing
- aerobics
- yoga

It is best to avoid exercise involving speed because Thyroid Types need more calming activities. However, I must admit I have a hard time following this suggestion. I love speeding along on my road bike, as well as going downhill or cross-country on my skis at a good clip. I also enjoy swimming, aerobics, and yoga occasionally. I believe the best exercise is the one that you love enough to do regularly. Pay attention to how it affects your energy levels and mood and make a change if it puts you in a negative frame of mind or depletes your energy for the rest of the day.

Vitamins and Supplements

Vitamins or dietary supplements can improve overall health and help manage some health conditions. Before you start any vitamin or supplement, **always** check with your physician and/or pharmacist to make sure that none of these supplements will worsen any pre-existing conditions or counteract with any of your existing medications.

Supplements typically most beneficial for Thyroid Types include:

- complex B: calms the nervous system
- vitamin C: supports the adrenal glands
- a protein digestive aid: for those who have trouble digesting protein or who are adding more protein into your diet, particularly if going back to eating more protein after being a vegetarian or vegan for years
- chromium: helps with sweet cravings
- spirulina: contains a powerful plant-based protein
- calcium magnesium: supports bones and maintains strength.
- protein supplements: Collagen or protein powder to help increase protein

Herbal Tea Suggestions

Raspberry leaf herbal tea naturally refreshes, and rosehip tea is a natural source of vitamin C that supports the adrenal glands.

Pituitary Type

Pituitary Type: The Quiet Thinking Type

There are few Pituitary Types, maybe only 5 percent of the population and most of them are men. With more than 80 percent of my clients being women, I have not encountered many.

If you look at the illustrations of the body types, you might think you're a Pituitary Type if you tend to gain weight all over your body. However, it's important to think back to when you started to gain weight. Maybe you first gained more weight in the upper body; if so, you may be an Adrenal Type. Or if you first gained weight in the lower body, you may be a Gonad Type. If you started by gaining weight all over your body, you may be a Pituitary Type.

Energy Levels: Morning Lark

The Pituitary Type is a morning person. Routinely getting up at five in the morning, they are tired at night. They also tend to need a nap or snack at 4 PM. Overall, though, they need very little sleep.

Personality Traits: Strategic Intellectual
with Plenty of Imagination

The pituitary is the gland of reason, the gland that regulates and creates stability. Pituitary Types are intellectuals with an active mind and a great deal of curiosity. They are the quiet thinking type with superior intellectual capacity. They tend to live in their head where they constantly reason, evaluate, analyze, compare, and judge. They also love to play strategic games, such as chess.

It would be good for them to learn how to calm the mental chatter at times.

Pituitary Types may be mathematicians, analysts, statisticians, actuaries, ambassadors, mediators, professors, or psychologists. They're also the philosopher: imaginative, reflective, calm, flexible, esoteric. Rather introverted, they are only sociable if others demand it. This can make them seem distant, even cold. They also tend to shy away from team sports. In fact, they may not care for sports at all. They are happier in their own world of imagination.

Pituitary Types also tend to have emotional insecurities. They reflect a long time before making any decision. They need a faithful partner, a stable relationship, and calm environment. They become exhausted by emotional discussions or confrontations, stressful situations like doctor appointments, and most any kind of manual labor or chores because they prefer to be in their heads. As a result,they can tend to eat when they are feeling emotional.

They need to get out of their head more often and feel, even welcome, their emotions. They need to challenge themselves to socialize and be more concerned about others.

If not careful, they tend to confront others without fearing a negative outcome. They also tend to act impulsively at times without analyzing the possible consequences first.

Nadia sounded young with a cheery voice when I talked with her on the phone. Five feet tall, she had always been slim at about 100 pounds. She emphasized that she wasn't thin and sickly looking when she was younger, but simply had a small build with thin bones. When she began gaining weight around the age of 35, it was soft baby-like fat, all over her body. Her neck became wider, her toes and fingers pudgier. At 46, she weighed 126 pounds and her body had become quite round. She didn't have the dairy cravings common among Pituitary Types because she didn't tolerate dairy products well. She did enjoy salty food and various types of tomato and creamy sauces, which made me think she might be an Adrenal or Gonad Type, but there was her personality...

Constantly analyzing everything, Nadia had difficulty making decisions. She often became emotional when struggling to make up her mind. When going through challenging times, she experienced indigestion as her system began to constrict with stress.

While growing up, she was expected to help in the grocery store her parents owned. She felt that she had missed out on her youth and was always seeking childlike activities to compensate, such as using her imagination to create fun games or play dress up with her kids.

Nadia had low blood sugar (hypoglycemia), so initially I asked her to follow the Thyroid Type plan, similar to the Pituitary Type plan in that it calls for quite a lot of protein at each meal. Pituitary Types feel much better if they are eating a diet high in protein. This was definitely the case with Nadia, who began feeling more balanced almost immediately. She also dropped the 20 pounds she had gained.

Now in her sixties, she easily maintains her ideal weight of 105 pounds, give or take a few, and delights in playing games and dress up with her grandchildren.

Physical Traits: Baby Face and a Round Frame

Pituitary Types usually have a baby face; they look younger than their age with very soft smooth skin. They have delicate hands and feet and fine hair. Pituitary Type women have small chests and buttocks. They also tend to have rounded shoulders with their head leaning slightly forward.

If they gain weight, it tends to be all over. The fat is soft, baby-like fat. They do not have much physical endurance and perspire a lot with minimal exertion.

Common Ailments: Respiratory Conditions

If Pituitary Types eat large quantities, they develop heartburn. Their digestion is good, but it tends to be slow at night.

The Pituitary Type often struggles with illnesses involving excess mucus because of an overconsumption of dairy products, which can increase mucus. When the body is irritated by something, it may produce additional or thicker mucus as protection against the irritating substance.

Pituitary Types are prone to allergies, colds, sinusitis, bronchitis, joint pain, and skin conditions such as psoriasis and eczema. Problems with the spinal column and shoulders are common, so it's important to stand and sit up straight to maintain good posture. They also tend not to have much interest in sex because they're happier being in their own head.

At four in the afternoon, Pituitary Type people need to eat or take a nap. They also tend to eat when they are feeling emotional.

Food Cravings: Dairy and Sweets

Pituitary Types often tend to be vegetarian. They don't care much for cooking and may think it's a waste of time. A meal could be as simple as reheating a bowl of soup or grabbing a sandwich.

Their cravings lean towards:

- dairy products, including ice cream;
- creamy sauces;
- honey;
- fruit;
- sorbet;
- cottage cheese;
- sugary sweets; and
- any food, such as cookies or toast, that can be accompanied by a glass of milk.

Note: It is important for everyone, but particularly Pituitary Types, to remember that even though you might crave dairy products, they may not agree with your body and result in excess mucus production. If you find your nose and/or throat often feeling stuffed up, opt for dairy alternatives for a few days to see if you are breathing easier or just feeling better.

Strategy for the Pituitary Type

Main Objective

Eating right for your body type will strengthen the adrenal and gonads (ovaries) without overstimulating the pituitary gland.

By reducing the dominance of the pituitary gland, your digestion will improve, which will help burn fat more rapidly. Your energy levels will be more stable throughout the day and your cravings will be reduced.

The foods that stimulate the adrenals the most include full proteins such as red meat and eggs. Chicken and fish are a little less stimulating, but they can be eaten for variety, as well as vegetarian protein such as tempeh, tofu, and beans.

Eliminate Dairy

The Pituitary Type's metabolism works a lot better without dairy products. The less dairy you consume, the better you will feel, as dairy may increase mucus in your respiratory system and also lead to weight gain.

Give up cream, milk, cheese, yogurt, and ice cream for a few weeks and see if you notice a difference, especially if you are trying to lose weight. Once you attain your desired weight, an occasional serving of organic yogurt is fine.

Eliminate Refined Carbohydrates, Simple Sugars, and Coffee

If you are trying to lose weight or just want to feel more balanced, remove white flour, white sugar, white rice, syrups, molasses, honey, brown sugar, coffee, tea, colas, and chocolate from your diet. Coffee and simple sugars overstimulate both the thyroid gland and the pituitary gland and leave you feeling off kilter.

Consume a 1/2 cup of healthy carbohydrates at each meal from whole, unrefined grains, whole stone-ground flours, such as buckwheat, millet, quinoa, spelt, Kamut Khorasan wheat, rye, brown rice, corn, or pasta made with whole-grain flours. Potatoes and fruit are also suitable carbohydrates. Two small pieces or servings of fruit per day are fine, so long as they are eaten before vegetables and the main course so the fruit can be more readily digested.

Eat Vegetables

Raw or cooked, enjoy these in abundance.

Meals Best Suited to Pituitary Type Energy

Large Breakfast Then Taper off through the Day

While for many people it is typical to eat a small breakfast, medium lunch, and a good-sized dinner, Pituitary Types need to reverse this pattern. The pituitary gland is very active, so your energy will be highest in the morning and almost inactive (low energy) at night. Breakfast should be copious (full protein such as eggs or meat), while lunch is a medium-sized meal and dinner is very light: a little fish, vegetarian protein such as legumes, or one egg.

Avoid Big, Late Dinners and Night Snacks

Pituitary Types have slow digestion at night, so late dinners can cause digestive problems. If your body is still digesting food when you go to bed, you will likely suffer from indigestion, insomnia, and gain weight.

Also, you need to be aware of your tendency to eat for emotional reasons. Beware of the nighttime snacks. You might ease the tension for a minute or two, but they will ultimately leave you feeling miserable.

The Pituitary Type Plan

Breakfast: Around 8 AM

Options

- eggs, soft boiled or poached (Eggs with runny yolks have less of an effect on cholesterol.)
- one slice of whole grain bread (Refer to the earlier section's notes about choosing good quality carbohydrates rather than refined ones.)
- healthy leftovers from the previous night's dinner, such as lean meat
- herbal tea: fenugreek and/or thyme (Read about their benefits in the herbal tea suggestions at the end of this chapter.)

Lunch: A Maximum of Four Hours after Breakfast

- a small piece or serving of fruit (It is best to have this before the meal so that the fruit is more easily digested.)

Vegetable Options

- a large salad (fresh vegetables, sprouts) with one tablespoon homemade dressing made with extra virgin olive oil or a cold-pressed vegetable oil
- a light, fat-free vegetable soup
- as many raw or cooked vegetables as you want

Carbohydrate Options

- a half a cup of healthy carbohydrates (brown rice, quinoa, barley, millet, potatoes, beans, pasta made from buckwheat, soy, spelt, Kamut Khorasan wheat, corn, or legumes)

- one slice of whole grain bread, preferably Kamut Khorasan wheat, spelt, or rye

Protein Options

- 4 to 6 oz of fish
- 4 oz of chicken (white meat)
- 4 oz of Tempeh or tofu, which are high in protein, or ½ to 1 cup lentils, chickpeas, kidney beans, or other kinds of beans

Optional Herbal Teas

- fenugreek and/or thyme

Dinner: A Maximum of Six Hours after Lunch

- a small piece or serving of fruit (which is important to have before the meal so that its fiber is better digested)

Vegetable Options

- a light, fat-free vegetable soup
- as many raw and/or cooked vegetables as you want

Protein Options

- 2 oz of fish or tofu
- 1 egg (poached or soft-boiled with the yolk runny so that it has less of an effect on cholesterol)

Carbohydrate Options

- a ½ cup of healthy carbohydrates (brown rice, quinoa, barley, millet, potatoes, beans, pasta made from buckwheat, soy, spelt, Kamut Khorasan wheat, corn, or legumes)

Optional extras

- ½ cup of yogurt (occasionally)

- 1 cup of skim milk, if tolerated (occasionally)
- herbal tea: fenugreek and/or thyme

Other Suggestions for the Pituitary Type

Get out of Your Head

Work in Pomodoro-type intervals and then take 'body breaks' in between. Dance to a favorite piece of music or get outside and take a walk in nature.

Take Care of Your Spine

Be mindful of your posture. Practising yoga helps with this.

Moisturize

Your skin tends to get dry, so lotions, oils, and creams are a good idea. Be mindful of the ingredients, though, as many lotions contain chemicals, check out the Skin Deep Database created by the Environmental Working Group for safe brands.

Get Your Game On

Your type tends to overthink things, so activities like walking and jogging aren't ideal because they allow for too much thinking. Instead, get a little more competitive and try activities that require your full attention. Ironically, you'll give your mind a break. Here are some ideas:

- aerobics with a predetermined routine
- karate
- t'ai chi
- ping pong, badminton, pickleball, etc.
- yoga

Vitamins and Supplements

Pituitary types absolutely need supplements that nourish the pituitary gland and the adrenals, because by stimulating the adrenals your type may be able to burn fat more efficiently and allow you to feel stronger and less inclined to snack. Always check with your physician and/or pharmacist to make sure that none of these supplements counteract with any of your existing medications.

- Calcium and magnesium with vitamin D bolster the pituitary gland.
- Alfalfa nourishes the pituitary gland.
- Vitamin C strengthens the adrenals.
- Spirulina nourishes the adrenals.
- Plant-based digestive enzymes help the hydrochloric acid in your stomach digest foods more efficiently.

Herbal Tea Suggestions

Fenugreek, known as nature's phlegm-buster, helps the respiratory system if you have extra mucus in your body from too much dairy. Thyme also helps the respiratory system, as well as being good for the digestive system on its own or in tandem with the fenugreek.

Part Three

Some Helpful Tips before Heading to the Grocery Store

Time for a Pantry Makeover

Congratulations! You have your body-type plan and you're ready to take your healthy eating to a whole new level! By learning how to replace unhealthy, filler food with more nutritionally dense alternatives, you will nourish your body and feel less hungry. You'll remain satiated longer, which will reduce the unhealthy snacking that can affect your weight.

Take some time to go through your pantry and fridge, cleaning out the unhealthy foods. Shop the sales and bulk items to find the foods you need. Healthier food often does cost more, but...

1. It's so nutrient dense that a little goes a long way so you can eat less of it and feel full longer.

2. You'll save money by buying less packaged, processed, refined, takeout, and restaurant food.

3. Your health is your most precious gift and the best investment you can make.

Healthy Grains and Carbs

Before heading to the store, shopping list in hand, let's learn why healthy carb choices are so much better for you.

Whole grains are high in fiber, low in calories, rich in minerals and vitamins, especially B vitamins. B vitamins nourish the nervous system, calming it, which helps you to better handle stress. Grains are also high in vitamin E, the anti-aging vitamin with its antioxidants. Healthy carbohydrates also give us more sustained, long-lasting energy.

Many people think that all grains or all carbohydrates are bad. Nothing could be further from the truth!

The primary mistake people make is in not distinguishing between good healthy grains and unhealthy refined grains. Often it is not the food that is unhealthy, but the way that it has been processed or prepared.

My clients are happy that they don't have to deprive themselves of carbs.

Let's Look at Refined Grains...

Grains are refined to lengthen their shelf life, which is important for the food industry. White and brown bread, pastries, cookies, crackers, and other 'baked' goods must last a long time in their packaging for most companies to profit.

When wheat is milled into flour, from 25 to 90 percent of the vitamins and minerals are lost, along with about half of the healthy fats. Much of the nutritional value is lost, and the flour is devoid of fiber. White flour is often bleached using a chemical whitening process involving chlorine gas. This may be linked to asthma and certain cancers. The process has been banned in Canada, Australia, and Europe.

When you eat products containing refined grains, you are consuming empty calories void of any nutrients. These foods will leave you feeling hungry and likely eating more — and often it's more of the same refined carbohydrates and sugars. Refined grains spike your blood sugar levels instantly, leaving you with the ensuing energy crash.

Now Let's Consider Healthy Grains

Healthy grains are whole grains. For instance, white rice has been polished to remove the outer layer with the healthy bran and germ, while brown rice still has these intact, which accounts for its brown color. If your breakfast cereal or bread has had its grain pulverized and processed into another form, the whole grain is no longer distinguishable.

Healthy whole grains include

- brown rice,
- quinoa,
- barley (scotch or pot barley is less refined than pearled, which has been polished),
- millet,
- buckwheat,
- rye, and
- oats.

When choosing bread, cereal, or pasta, be sure they are made with the grains mentioned above, or also...

- Kamu Khorasan wheat,
- spelt,
- organic, non-genetically modified (GMO) soy, or
- organic, non-GMO corn.

What About Wheat?

Over the years, wheat has been modified and manipulated. Sometimes the seeds are treated with insecticides, fungicides, and growth regulators. When my clients switch from regular wheat to healthier grain alternatives, such as Kamut Khorasan wheat, or spelt, they tell me their bloating disappears.

If you do eat wheat on occasion, look for bread that is stone ground. When grains are ground using metal blades, the heat removes the germ that contains most of the grain's nutrients.

It's important to note that breads and pasta may be described as whole wheat on the package, but that doesn't necessarily mean the whole grain is being used. Only part of the grain is incorporated in some cases, and this refined wheat might have less nutritional value. A healthier choice is 100% whole grain and should be described as such on the package.

White rice, like white flour, is less nutritionally dense. When the rice is polished, the bran part, where we find all the minerals and B vitamins, is removed. Brown rice and whole grains were once eaten around the world. Then it became fashionable for rich people to have rice and bread that was made white by workers, who polished the grains by hand. Wanting to emulate the rich, the Industrial Revolution's emergent working class sought refined grains, unknowingly making everyone poorer health-wise. Some people ask if basmati rice is better; it is simply a different kind of rice. You can buy brown basmati rice.

Let's Go Shopping!

Okay! Let's stock your pantry, fridge, and freezer with healthy food. Keeping it handy will help set you up by having everything you need to grab for healthy snacks and easy-to-prepare meals.

It may take a bit of time for you to source your new healthy choices. You might be lucky enough to have a health food or grocery store that stocks organic produce and nutrient dense carbs and proteins. But you might also have to go out of your way to connect with local farmers or even shop online — especially if you live in a small community. If you're not signed up for a farmer's basket, choose what's in season at your grocery store whenever possible.

Fruits and Vegetables: Prep for a Better Experience

Starting with the fruit and vegetable section, I buy what looks fresh and is preferably on sale. Buy your favorites in abundance. You're aiming to fill half your plate with vegetables at lunch and at dinner.

Once you get your groceries home, start using the veggies that wilt quickly, such as the dark leafy greens. Dark leafy green vegetables are known to be highest in nutrient density. Green inside means clean inside. In other words, you also help the body to detoxify.

Wash, dry, and chop up the parsley, cilantro and other tender-leaf herbs and keep them in small containers in the fridge so you can readily add them to dishes.

Turnips, beets, potatoes, and other root vegetables last the longest.

It's normal for those of us living in cold climates to gravitate more toward lighter salads and raw vegetables in summer and to soups and heartier vegetables that are steamed or cooked during the winter.

I am fortunate to live just outside Montreal where large health food stores abound. My main go-to vegetables in the winter are kale and Swiss chard. When kale is fresh, I massage it with homemade salad dressing, which softens it. Fast and easy, and high in fiber, kale is one of the most nutrient-dense foods you can buy. If it starts to get a little limp, I sauté onion and garlic in butter and olive oil and stir in pieces of kale. Then I add a little water, cover, and braise it until soft and served with lemon juice. This is a delicious recipe for all dark leafy greens, such as Swiss chard, beet greens, or rapini.

Swiss chard looks like huge spinach leaves with thick bright red or yellow stems. The large leaves make it so much easier to clean than spinach and it takes only a few minutes to steam.

Stock up on lemons to squeeze on top of your dark leafy greens to add flavour and vitamin C.

Celery and carrots are two other staples I always have on hand. Celery is high in organic sodium as well as digestive enzymes, making it perfect to munch before a meal. One of my clients was astounded when her acid reflux disappeared by eating celery before dinner. She told all her friends and family that they should do the same. Of course, it's not a miracle cure, but can help.

On weekends, when my partner and I celebrate happy hour with some beer or wine, we often have celery, carrots, and other veggies, such as red peppers or cauliflower, with homemade hummus. This is also the perfect appetizer when his kids come over for dinner or when we have a gathering with friends. The kaleidoscope of color looks beautiful, and everyone enjoys those added vegetables without filling up on something heavy like cheese and crackers or nachos before the meal. Note that red peppers pack the most nutrition, much higher than any of the other sweet pepper colors, especially in terms of vitamin C and beta-carotene.

In terms of other fresh vegetables, I integrate as much variety and color as possible each week: broccoli, cauliflower, beans, squash, turnip, tomatoes, mushrooms, bok choy, spinach, cabbage, and others. If you are busy, look for pre-cut or frozen vegetables.

Sugar: Not a Problem with Fruit and Carrots

I've had quite a few new clients tell me that they're steering away from fruit because of the high sugar content. They also believe that they should avoid carrots as they've heard that they are high on the glycemic index.

If it grows, it's typically good for you. If you have diabetes or a serious sugar addiction, then reducing your fruit consumption can help balance blood sugar and alleviate sweet cravings, but this isn't the case for most people. Buy fruit, preferably in season. It makes a perfect snack, especially when you're hungry and preparing dinner. This tip is helpful for those who tend to sample as they cook.

As for carrots, a diet high in vegetables has been linked to a lower risk of cardiovascular disease, cataracts, macular degeneration, cognitive decline, and digestive tract cancers. Carrots help reduce inflammation and boost immunity.

Best Snacks are Homemade Snacks

In health food stores, there are so-called 'healthy' snacks everywhere! I had one client tell me, "It said 'healthy' on the package!"

Please don't be fooled by misleading claims. Steer clear of packaged chips, cookies, and crackers. Healthy crackers to grab are Ryvita, Kavli, and brown rice cakes. Keep on pushing your cart past everything else.

Instead, as much as possible, make your own or stock up on ingredients for trail mix in the dried fruit and nut section.

My 4 go-to snacks are:

1. My sensational homemade power bars: See the recipe section on p.129 or online at https://www.bodytypology.com/protein-bar-recipe.html.

2. Trail mix: Create your own with the tips below and see the recipe section on p.136.

3. Fruit: Those who are hypoglycemic or diabetic should include a little protein such as nuts or nut butter to keep their blood sugar balanced.

4. Veggies with homemade hummus (See the recipe section p.144 or online at https://www.bodytypology.com/hummus-recipe. html.)

The bulk bins are the perfect place to stock up on the power bar ingredients and everything you'll need for trail mix. Buy natural organic raisins as other raisins may be coated in unhealthy vegetable oils to keep them from sticking together. Dried apricots are a delicious choice. They should be brown. Bright orange ones have been treated with sulfites. Dates are another healthy snack that some people mistakenly think is too high in sugar.

Almonds or walnuts are a good choice, but not too many if you'd like to drop some pounds. Make sure they're plain, not salted or roasted, because fats are healthier in their raw state. Sunflower seeds and pumpkin seeds are other great additions to your trail mix. Goji berries, which look similar to raisins but are red, are packed with nutrients and antioxidants. Combining your own ingredients into a trail mix is worth it as the packaged ones usually contain roasted nuts, added salt, unhealthy oils, and sugar-coated foods.

Peanuts are grown in a humid climate. Even the organic ones can have aflatoxins, a type of mold that makes them hard on the liver. For this reason, almond butter is a better choice than peanut butter.

Watch Out for Unnecessary Additives in Condiments

Health food stores generally stock healthier condiments, such as soy sauce, so you can make your own sauces and salad dressings to avoid the unnecessary sugar, salt, preservative chemicals, and food coloring.

That's why we're swinging by the store's oil and vinegar section, which is key to help you steer clear of bottled salad dressings. Choose a good quality extra virgin olive oil, an organic first cold-pressed oil such as sunflower or canola, as well as some grape seed oil, which has a lower smoke point and is therefore better when heated to a high temperature. Toasted sesame seed oil adds a delicious flavor to Asian type sauces. An easy, basic salad dressing is one-part vinegar to two-parts oil. Add in your sea salt from France (Celtic, grey in color, is best) and any other ingredients you wish, such as dried basil, oregano, or Dijon mustard.

In keeping with the principle that food in its most natural state is best, buy unpasteurized vinegars whenever possible. Any flavor is fine: red wine, balsamic, rice, or apple cider vinegar.

You may have read articles touting apple cider vinegar as the miracle cure for just about everything, including weight loss, but unfortunately, these are generally exaggerated claims. The main benefit is that good quality unpasteurized apple cider vinegar mimics the hydrochloric acid in our stomach. People under the age of thirty with a lot of anxiety tend to produce a lot of hydrochloric acid, so adding in extra apple cider vinegar could make this worse. As we age, our stomach tends to produce less hydrochloric acid, so apple cider vinegar can aid digestion. Some people enjoy taking a teaspoon of it in a little water with a meal and notice an improvement in their digestion. Everyone has different tastes. I enjoy it in homemade salad dressing but don't care for it on its own.

Bragg is a brand name that makes excellent unpasteurized apple cider vinegar. I also recommend Bragg Liquid Aminos. Adrenal Types, along with some Gonad Types who tend to enjoy salt, love this soy sauce. Made with only soybeans and water, it contains none of the added sugar, coloring or chemical preservatives found in most soy sauces. This can be a game changer for your family to enjoy food they usually turn their noses up at. It's delicious on top of vegetables or healthy carbs such as brown rice and quinoa.

I also prefer to buy mayonnaise, Dijon mustard, and other condiments in the health food store because the products typically contain fewer and healthier ingredients. I make a delicious, sugar-free ketchup using a base of tomato paste and herbs. See recipe p. 141 and website: https://www.bodytypology.com/heart-healthy-recipes.html.

Herbs and Spices Can Be Purchased in Any Store.

I encourage you to grow a few of your own every spring. Even if you live in an apartment or condominium, you can keep a few pots of fresh herbs to add to salads and other dishes. Every year I grow basil, mint and parsley from seed or small plants. Experiment to find what grows best in your space.

Eat Your Beans

According to *The Journal of Nutrition*, 96 percent of Americans don't meet the minimum daily recommended amounts of legumes, also known as beans or pulses. This is the same percentage of Americans who don't eat enough dark green vegetables. Legumes and dark leafy greens are two of the healthiest foods on the planet!

Nutrient rich, super economical, high in fiber and protein, it's time to make beans a part of your healthy diet.

When I first became vegetarian, I struggled with consuming enough healthy protein. I ate too much cheese and processed pseudo-meat products instead.

Beans are a much healthier choice. A serving of beans costs between 10 and 40 cents. Most canned beans contain 100 percent more sodium than home-cooked. Draining and rinsing will only remove 45 to 50 percent of the sodium, so buy unsalted whenever possible or prepare your own.

I always buy dried beans, soak them overnight, throw out the soaking water, then cook them. This is a great task to do on the weekend while doing something else at home. During cooking, leave the lid off slightly to allow the gases to escape. This makes them more digestible and less likely to cause gas when they are eaten. I freeze them in two-cup portions and defrost them as needed.

Canned beans are pressure cooked in the can, which causes them to create more gas when eaten. If you haven't been eating a lot of legumes, start off with small portions and gradually increase over time to allow your body to adjust. This way you are less like to suffer from gas.

Stock up on all kinds of beans to benefit from the different nutrients each one provides, as well as the different colors, textures, and flavors.

What To Use for Sweetener?

Moving on to the baking section, grab a bottle of liquid stevia. I like the plain, organic *Now* brand. If you are looking at other brands, check the ingredients. They should include only stevia extract, water, and alcohol as a preservative. Stay away from the flavored stevia.

My partner switched from sugar to stevia to sweeten his coffee. He bought a bottle of liquid stevia that had "pure" in its name, along with a description as a zero-calorie liquid sweetener. Should be good, right? The second ingredient after water was erythritol, a sugar alcohol. It also contained the chemical preservatives sodium benzoate and potassium sorbate.

If you enjoy baking, perhaps choose xylitol or raw sugar. Other good natural sweeteners include unpasteurized honey and pure maple syrup.

I often replace or reduce the amount of sweetener in dessert recipes. I also switch the type of flour to make my own healthier version, usually using Kamut Khorasan wheat or spelt flour.

High Quality Protein Sources

Stock up on your favorite kinds of protein. I buy organic eggs that are from free-range chickens because the quality seems to be better and more satiating. You may come across two descriptors for eggs: 'cage-free' and 'free range'. The difference is that free range hens generally have access to some form of outside area, though there are no standards for how long hens have access or what the outdoor access is like.

For lunch, I generally choose a vegetarian protein, often beans or lentils and occasionally tempeh, or tofu.

Dinner can be fish, organic chicken, or another vegetarian protein. I often roast two organic chickens and make bone broth the next day. I prefer the taste and texture of organic chickens that are fed an organic diet, not one maximized for growth.

I often get asked about tofu or tempeh, which is similar to tofu. Neither have much flavor. You need to marinate them, preferably overnight. Both are high in protein, with tempeh being the vegetarian food that is highest in protein.

It was once thought that eating soy-based solids could increase the risk of breast cancer, but now studies show the opposite is true. I suggest you do your own research and always choose soy products that are organic and non-GMO. Tempeh is found in the freezer section of most stores.

High Quality Carbs

Your last stop is the bread aisle. I get my brown rice and Kamut Khorasan wheat flour for baking in the bulk section. If you don't have access to bulk bins, these are usually sold alongside the bags of oats, quinoa, and barley.

I wish that Kamut Khorasan wheat or spelt sourdough bread would be readily available globally, because I find it is the most nutrient dense, healthy bread. Unfortunately, we are nowhere near there yet. If you're able to get Kamut Khorasan wheat flour, perhaps you could make some bread in a bread-making machine. Or have pasta made with Kamut Khorasan wheat instead. If you don't have those choices, I suggest rye bread.

Note: while refined white flour can last for years in the pantry, whole flours are best refrigerated because they can go rancid more quickly.

If you are gluten-free, the challenge is the breads you can eat are usually high in sugar. It's probably best to kick the bread habit and choose other carbs for lunch and dinner: brown rice, quinoa, potatoes, or sweet potatoes.

Congrats on Investing in Your Health

Okay, it's time to take a deep breath and head to the cash. You know that your full basket of healthy food is going to cost a lot more than your usual less expensive fare. However, with the healthier food you are buying, a little goes a long way! You'll feel full having a smaller amount and you'll feel satisfied a lot longer. And it's worth the investment to feel better too. Your health is the most precious gift of this journey. The choices you make today affect your quality of life tomorrow. You're worth the investment. Good for you for prioritizing your health!

What Can Hinder Weight Loss?

Some of my new clients are worried that Bodytopology might not work for them when it comes to losing weight. They ask me if I have had some clients for whom the program hasn't been successful.

In general, eating right for your body type will help you drop excess weight. That said, a few of my clients haven't been able to lose weight.

Most often, it's because they've lacked the motivation to follow their body type's plan or didn't exercise regularly.

Here are some other circumstances that can slow, even stall, weight loss:

Hypothyroidism

Besides weight gain, some of the signs of an underactive thyroid include

- feeling cold, especially in the evening;
- cold hands and feet, especially in the evening;
- hair loss;
- dry skin;
- fatigue;
- depression; and
- getting upset for minor reasons.

A simple blood test can confirm low thyroid function.

Stress

Stress exacerbates most health issues. When the body is stressed, it may gain or hold on to weight. You may be eating larger amounts or eating more often to calm your nerves. Chronic stress may increase the rate at which fat cells are formed, according to research featured in *The Cell Metabolism Journal*.

A simple remedy: When I taught yoga, I would constantly remind my students to bring their awareness back to focus on their deep abdominal breathing. I think this simple practice is the most beneficial thing you can do to reduce a stress response.

Trauma and Negative Emotions

When I was studying to become a naturopath, my teacher said that for the body to release weight, energy must flow. She meant that there needs to be a sense of joy or love, or purpose, resulting in the creation and release of positive emotions and energy. At the time, I didn't fully understand why that flow was essential. As I continued to build my practice and advise more clients, I better understood what my teacher meant when she asked: "Is there love in your life?"

- love of self
- love of your life
- love of the people around you
- love of where you live
- love of where you work and what you do
- love of children
- love of pets/animals
- love of volunteering/being of service

If you believe that emotions are a kind of energy that flows through the body, then perhaps someone who is holding onto negative emotions, such as resentment, anger, or bitterness, could have energy that is stuck. And that might hinder weight loss.

Monique, who had been sexually abused when she was young, kept holding onto a lot of anger. She seemed to be following her Adrenal Type plan closely, but week after week, her weight remained the same even after following the program for three months. Processing and releasing some of that anger through therapy might have helped.

A Congested Liver

Years ago, while my osteopath was bending my leg by pushing it against my abdomen, I felt some pain. When I asked her what might be causing it, she said my liver was congested. I was surprised as I thought that by following a healthy diet and exercising regularly, my liver would be fine. She explained that many people have a liver that could use some additional support. Those of us living in urban areas are breathing in more air pollution. We are also exposed to chemicals and/or toxins in our household, beauty, and cleaning products, as well as flame retardants on materials such as carpets, curtains and upholstery.

The liver has many functions, including filtering toxins from the body. When the liver is overworked due to a diet high in fat or excess alcohol, or an overexposure to chemicals, it gets congested and cannot process sugars and fats as effectively, causing fat to build up in other parts of the body, hence weight gain.

Dietician Kristin Kirkpatrick and hepatologist Ibrahim Hanouneh have some suggestions for showing your liver a little more love in their book, *Skinny Liver*. They include

- reducing alcohol intake,
- getting adequate, good quality sleep,
- managing stress,
- maintaining a healthy weight,
- exercise, and
- following a healthy diet.

Certain Medications

There are some medications that increase appetite or cause water retention and weight gain as their side effects. Antidepressants and antipsychotic drugs may slow down the body and its metabolism, which can stall weight loss. I have had success with clients who have been on antidepressants, but the progress is slower due to the medication.

Restrictive Diets

New clients often ask me how fast they can expect to drop the pounds. Everyone is different — there is no set norm. My primary goal is to encourage people to learn a healthy way of eating that is best for their particular body type with a regimen they can follow for the rest of their life. It is my experience that excess weight tends to come off in the majority of cases. You're also more likely to keep that weight off by continuing to eat right for your body type.

Many clients lose weight more quickly at the beginning, especially if they have been eating an unhealthy diet. After a while, the weight loss tapers off to a pound or two per week. This is a healthy rate that is more likely to lead to sustained, long-term weight loss.

Research indicates that an overly restrictive diet can actually slow down your metabolism and lead to more weight gain as soon as the diet ends or is adjusted to be sustainable longer term.

Someone who has done a lot of yo-yo dieting in the past might lose weight more slowly when they start eating for their body type. But if you don't start seeing results after a few weeks, you might want to re-read the description of the body types to ensure you have the right plan.

Be As Healthy as You Can and Follow Your Plan

I realize some of the circumstances I have mentioned are not within your control, but I believe that the healthier you are overall, the easier it will be for you to drop the pounds you want to drop.

Know also that as you increase your exercise, muscle is denser than fat, so you might not see a rapid change on the scale. You will see the difference in your clothes; when your long-time favourite jeans, for instance, no longer feel as if they have been spray-painted onto your legs.

You should begin seeing results after a few weeks, and the more closely you follow your body type's plan, the faster the changes in your body will happen.

Long-Term Healing

Whenever I start working with a new client, I always talk about the four pillars of health:

1. Diet

2. Exercise

3. Supplements and vitamins

4. Healthy lifestyle, environment, and outlook

I discuss the first three in terms of each body type in the earlier chapters of this book. A healthy lifestyle, environment, and outlook can involve everything from establishing ways to minimize and/or manage stress, choosing natural, chemical-free skincare and cleaning products, to being around positive, like-minded people.

Working with people's mindsets is where I spend a lot of my coaching time with clients. Soon after I began my practice, I realized that while following their body type diet could transform the health and lives of my clients, these positive changes might be short-lived unless I found a way to help them heal the emotional causes of their excess weight and/or physical ailments. I also realized that many people were unaware of how big a role emotional eating played in their unhealthy habits. Without help with this aspect of their lifestyle, they might revert to their old way of eating to manage stressful situations, then regain the weight, become discouraged, and feel like they'd failed.

Therapy, combined with decades of soul-searching through workshops and self-help books, helped me get to a healthier, happier place in my life. I wondered if I could I do more for my clients at this deeper level without sending them for years of therapy.

A friend suggested I look into Rapid Transformational Therapy (RTT). I've always been fascinated by how the mind works, so I signed up for the course and immediately loved the material.

Hypnosis is effective because it allows people to quiet the analytical and intellectual chatter in the mind and more easily focus on what is deeper down and more important to them. Capri Cruz, Ph.D., psychotherapist and hypnotherapist and author of *Maximize Your Super Powers* says, "hypnosis addresses the cause and other contributing factors directly at the subconscious level in the person's mind, where their memories, habits, fears, food associations, negative self-talk, and self-esteem germinate. No other weight loss method addresses the core issues at the root like hypnosis does."

Marisa Peer, RTT's world-renowned founder, has been successfully practicing it in England for more than 30 years and has won numerous awards for developing a method using hypnotherapy combined with unique techniques for long-lasting results. RTT can be effective in overcoming emotional eating, breaking unhealthy habits, increasing self-esteem, alleviating fears and phobias, and resolving childhood trauma.

In the conscious mind, we often stay stuck in a familiar loop of emotions where logical willpower doesn't work.

Using hypnotherapy, we access the subconscious mind where the experiences that shape how we feel and why we react in a particular way are stored, as if in a vault. We uncover key memories and work through them and then plant, like seeds, positive suggestions in the subconscious mind. The new beliefs take root. RTT has been designed to provide rapid relief and permanent results in as little as one to three sessions.

Marisa reiterated what I believed to be true for a long time: most people suffer from a lack of self-worth. They feel like they're not enough and until they change this, success in any area of their lives will be hindered.

During the course, the students practiced on each other, and I became more confident with each session. As soon as I graduated, I began using RTT with my clients and my success rate soared.

One of the questions I ask my clients is what life will look like *without* the problems they mention on their intake forms. I take notes and expand on their answers to create a powerful, positive script. After doing the RTT process to discover, release and reframe what's been holding them back,

I prepare and record a script with positive suggestions that are unique to that client's needs. I ask the client to listen to the recording daily for 21 consecutive days. One of the rules of the mind is that your brain is wired to keep returning to what is familiar. With the recording we make the familiar unfamiliar, and the unfamiliar familiar.

Chloe was a shy, Gonad Type mom of three who had trouble asking for help. After an RTT session, she enjoyed dancing at parties, found a higher paying job and insisted that her husband make her some chicken soup when she had a cold.

Vivian, who tended to be stuck in critical internal chatter, said it was as if I had removed a negative black wire from her brain and inserted a positive white one instead.

Another client realized during her RTT session that after her miscarriage, she began to use food to try to fill a void in her soul.

Recognizing these catalytic moments and replacing the thinking patterns they create with a more positive mind set and thought pattern is key to the necessary healing for our long-term success.

What thoughts and beliefs are you ready to release? Write them down and recast them into positive mantras to say every day.

If you find you are using food to suppress your emotions or fill a void in your life, you might want to find a RTT practitioner or other qualified therapist.

Emotional Eating

Virtually all of us, at some time, have been hurt or disappointed and suppressed those feelings. In my case, I was angry at my dad for leaving our family when I was young. I was angry at my mom for being overly controlling and guilt-tripping.

During my 20s and 30s, I was stuck in a waitressing job I loathed, and wanting to meet someone special, yet always choosing the wrong kind of guy....

Instead of food, my chosen weapons of numbing were alcohol, marijuana, and excessive work. The psychologist I was dating when I was 40 encouraged me to do weekly therapy sessions for a year. With help, I started allowing some of those stuffed down emotions to surface and be released.

I had no idea I had buried so much pain, sadness, and anger. I cried my heart out and projected a lot of my rage onto my boyfriend. Thank goodness he was a psychologist and didn't take it personally.

By the end of the year, I felt lighter, happier, more self-confident. My boyfriend said I was no longer the same person.

I believe that shedding tears is one of the most beneficial ways to release long-held anger or pain. Tears heal the heart. When we allow a long-buried emotion to surface and we spend time consciously feeling and processing it, we can usually release it forever. That is when real transformation occurs.

Janet, one of my Gonad Type clients, told me that her parents never showed her love. There were rarely any hugs or other kinds of affection displayed. When Janet was young, her parents also told her they couldn't afford anything beyond their basic needs.

She wished she could play soccer with her girlfriends, but that was considered an unnecessary expense.

Janet had planned a July 2020 wedding. After lengthy discussions with her fiancé, they decided to postpone it for a year because of COVID-19. Janet shed more than a few tears about the delay. When she informed her mother about the decision, there was no attempt to console her.

"Just postpone the damn wedding!" was all her mother said.

Janet immediately craved a glass of wine.

Rather than feeling challenging emotions, we often reach for a glass of wine or some junk food.

We live in a society that advocates that we should always be happy. And there is no end to the distractions we can use to keep us from feeling our emotions: food, drugs, alcohol, sex, work, shopping, streaming TV programs, social media... All of these provide an escape but it's temporary.

Nancy was a 55-year-old Adrenal Type who consulted with me over three months. On her health intake form, she mentioned she suffered from depression, a mood disorder, an eating disorder (binging on sweets), insomnia, and an inability to focus. She also had arthritis, recurrent urinary tract infections, and a fatty liver. Her food journal indicated that she ate a lot of sweets, in addition to skipping meals and grabbing unhealthy restaurant food on the go.

I had her follow her Adrenal Type plan and do a sugar detox. She loved her workout classes at the gym, an excellent outlet.

During her second session, Nancy said her son had told his therapist that his mom played 'the victim'. This upset her, but she acknowledged there was some truth to it.

The following session, I suggested that she be aware of using the words *don't*, *not* and *no*. I encouraged her to change her negative vocabulary into positive words. She also began listening to a meditation app to better manage her stress.

Over the weeks together, we identified things for her to do instead of indulging in sweet cravings, such as having an herbal tea, moving her body, or journaling. I also had her do writing exercises to build her self-esteem. She began recognizing her pattern of wanting sweets whenever she felt unhappy, so she made a conscious effort to stop using food to avoid sad or bad moods. She listened to motivating audio books, including one about cognitive behavior therapy.

After nine sessions, she noticed that her arthritic pain was gone.

That same week, her boss talked to her about her attitude, saying there had been complaints from a few employees that she was often negative. His delivery was harsh. She was devastated. At a subsequent company-related conference, she remained in her room most of the time, crying for hours. The following week, however, she told her boss that he lacked tact in the way he had talked to her. She also shared a bit about the challenges that she was facing. Her boss apologised, and she felt empowered by speaking up for herself.

During our final session, I realized that the woman in front of me was not the same one who had originally come to see me. Nancy had quit her sugar addiction and was eating healthy, balanced meals. She lost 12 pounds and 5½ inches off her chest, waist, and hips. She was energetic and self-confident. She told me the work she had done during our time together had been life-changing.

I followed up with her a few months later. She was finding it challenging with all the gyms closed because of COVID-19. She missed the workouts that gave her both a physical and emotional release. She had kept most of her other healthy habits, but a few bad ones had returned. She had gained some of the weight back and still found herself struggling with emotional eating occasionally. But this time she had some victories under her belt too.

Healing emotional wounds and undoing the old habits created by them can be challenging to work through on your own. Plus, healing is not a linear process. There are bound to be ups and downs. It's important to give yourself permission to heal slowly and honor yourself for working through the feelings, knowing that two steps forward and one step back is still forward.

Carolyn was 19 when she contacted me. Her dad had come across my program and suggested that she inquire about it. She was a high-achieving, studious Adrenal Type who wanted to be a psychologist. She said she wanted to learn how to control her mind and body.

As I spoke with her, it quickly became apparent to me that she was dating someone who was disrespectful. They often argued, which left her feeling angry and hurt. When, during a session, Carolyn told me that she'd had yet another huge fight with her boyfriend and had decided to simply be with her anger and sadness, I knew we were making progress. In the past, she would have reached for ice cream or chips to comfort herself. This time she rode the wave of emotions and found that the feelings passed after a while. She learned that she didn't have to turn to food because bad feelings don't last forever.

I wanted to shout "halleluiah" from the rooftops! At 19, Carolyn had learned what many people never realize: that we can resist the urge to turn to food or other numbing distractions and instead allow ourselves the time to be with an uncomfortable feeling until it passes. And it will pass.

Carolyn dropped 35 pounds over the next six months and eventually dumped her boyfriend.

Becoming Aware of Emotional Triggers

The first step towards bringing about real change is awareness. It's essential to become familiar with your daily life patterns. Sometimes we don't even realize how often we're doing something unhealthy until we make note of it. Erin was a young client who was challenged with a lot of anxiety and stress that would cause her to reach for food. She recognized early on that her cravings were emotional and chose to play with her puppy instead.

Keep an Emotional Eating Food Journal

Jot down, in a journal, all your eating behaviors for a full week. Don't try to change anything. Just keep track of everything. Instead of counting calories or food points as some weight-loss programs suggest, write down what time it was, what exactly you ate, some indication of the amount, what was happening immediately before you ate and, most importantly, how you were feeling — the emotion connected to that food — before and after you ate, along with any other insights.

I've made a handy emotional eating chart for you to use:

https://www.bodytypology.com/book.html

Within days, you'll likely start to notice patterns. If you're honest with yourself, you'll see what's really behind some of your food decisions.

Reflect on what you are discovering: What feelings are you experiencing when you have the urge to eat, overeat, or consume junk food when you're not hungry? What triggers are driving your emotional hunger?

Here are some possibilities:

- Have you been depressed about something and using food to cope with the lows?
- Is your emotional eating triggered by a certain person: a difficult boss or co-worker, a rebellious teen, or another unhappy relative?
- Is your life-partner relationship strained and you're using food to distract yourself from arguments and unmet needs?
- Are you feeling there's something big missing in your life and you're compensating for this lack with food?
- Are you using food as a reward at the end of a difficult day or as stress management?
- Are your feelings triggered by events that happened when you were a child?

There may be some things that come up that you have been avoiding for a very long time. How has your emotional eating been serving you?

Note: Sometimes if there has been sexual abuse, an individual may unconsciously become and stay overweight so they don't attract any further unwanted attention from others. Some may feel that if they are bigger or stronger than others, they will not be bullied.

In short, emotional eating helps you to temporarily avoid the feelings you don't want to feel. Look at your list of emotional eating triggers and see what can and can't be changed. You may not be able to change your job right now, but maybe you can start making small steps towards finding other employment. Maybe you need to spend less time with a relative or friend who causes you to head for the fridge as soon as you arrive back home. Rank the items in order of the easiest to hardest to change. Make a step-by-step plan.

I realize some of the circumstances that I have mentioned that can hinder weight loss are not within your control, but I believe that the healthier you are overall, the easier it will be for you to drop the pounds you want gone. You should start seeing results after a few weeks and the more closely you follow your body type plan, the faster the weight loss will happen.

Overcoming self-criticism

A key question is: *Why did you gain weight?* Weight gain is often the result of a life imbalance. What needs to be rebalanced in your life? Can you remember what was happening in your life when you first started to put on pounds?

Love is at the heart of many problems... and solutions. Especially love of self. I firmly believe that for long-term success in maintaining a healthy weight, you must have a good sense of self-worth and a routine of self-care.

How do you love yourself if you grew up with frequent criticism rather than praise and encouragement? What is that inner voice saying to you throughout your day? Is much of it negative? It may seem like an impossible task to shift from chronic negativity to a more optimistic outlook, but let me assure you that it can be done.

It took me decades to establish my self-worth and self-confidence. The journey was challenging, but also interesting. Everything I did to push out of my comfort zone — traveling, going away to university, signing up for courses and mentorship, reading self-help books, therapy, learning yoga and meditation — all helped me.

Everybody's journey is different. As Marianne Williamson said, "And as we let our own light shine, we unconsciously give other people permission to do the same. As we're liberated from our own fear, our presence automatically liberates others."

And it may not need to take you decades. Sometimes it works to simply identify the root causes of self-inflicted negativity and then find a process to reframe, release, and replace that negativity with a more positive mindset.

Anne's family dynamics also led to her suffering from a lack of self-worth. Her father left when she was very young, trapping her with a physically and emotionally abusive mother. Anne fled home at 19 with only the clothes on her back and her laptop, never to return. She had to file a restraining order to protect herself from her mother.

Eventually she met someone special, moved to Montreal, married, and began classes to work in the travel industry. She was 25 years old when she came to see me for weight loss. As she gained weight, she felt she was starting to resemble her overweight mother, which she didn't want. She hadn't had any contact with her mother for five years.

In her sessions with me, Anne began doing a lot of inner work. Simply talking about her past seemed to help her feel better. When I complimented her, during the beginning of our sessions together, she tended to hide her face in her hands. I suggested she could let go of that, which she did.

I encourage my clients to choose their *core feelings* for each week — how they want to feel over the next seven days while working towards their goals. It is a practice encouraged by Danielle LaPorte in her book *Desire Map*.

At first, Anne chose words such as *light, centered, grounded,* and *at ease.* She was reading *Unleash the Power Within* by Tony Robbins.

As we began, Anne started to eat right for her body type and exercising. Her excess weight was coming off and a lot of her digestive ailments quickly disappeared.

During our fifth consultation, she chose *sexy* and *confident* as her core feelings and kept those for three weeks. She arrived at my office looking chic in new clothes, rocking with confidence. She said her family and friends were commenting on her new appearance, which made her feel great.

Even with her busy schedule of full-time work plus off-hours schooling,

Anne kept eating healthily. She also began doing things she had long wanted to try. She got a tattoo, and then a second. She took a course in burlesque dancing and entered a contest at a bar, getting up on stage to a roar of applause.

After 12 sessions, Anne had lost 15 pounds.

"I am being more direct and honest and just *me*. I'm focusing on myself and my life, instead of trying to get approval from everyone else, she said."

Anne realized that a lot of her weight gain was related to self-sabotage that came from thinking she was never good enough. As she learned how to follow her body type's plan, she had a lot more energy, better handled her stress, and was having *aha* moments every day.

We worked together for a further twelve sessions, and she achieved a weight that felt right for her. She continued to develop more self-assurance and self-confidence. She easily handled matters that would have bothered her in the past, such as conflict with her boss.

After five years of no contact with her mother, Anne talked to her that Christmas. Her mother sent her a box with some of her requested belongings as well as some unexpected gifts. Their relationship improved and Anne has become determined to no longer be held hostage by it, no matter how it evolves.

Transforming Negative Thoughts

In working with numerous clients, I've come to realize that healthy eating is more about the thoughts we put in our heads than the food we put in our mouths.

Say what?

Of course, eating right for your body type is the most effective way to achieve and maintain your ideal weight. However, long-term success also requires examining what ideas you're repeatedly feeding your brain. Our thoughts ultimately dictate what we eat, as well as how much and how often, along with how much alcohol we consume, and whether or not we exercise.

So many of us can be hard on ourselves. When struggling with either overeating or eating unhealthy food, it's easy to fall into a lot of negative self-talk to the point of self-loathing, even self-hatred.

"There is only one thing I ever work on with anyone and this is loving the self," Louise Hay wrote in her book, *You Can Heal Your Life*. " Love is the miracle cure. Loving ourselves works miracles in our lives."

We need to make a full stop to examine how we are mentally beating ourselves up and why. We then need to re-cast that negative self-talk into positive affirmations and read or say them to ourselves every time we catch ourselves reverting back to those old negative thoughts. Those are well-worn neural pathways, but our brains are nimble. Just like working with weights develops our muscular strength, working with affirmations develops a stronger, happier mind.

I grew up with a lot of negativity and developed a pattern of constantly criticizing myself, which would spiral into moods of worry and despair.

I started to flip that pattern with Clint Best, an awesome business coach I worked with for a year while teaching yoga and building my practice as a naturopath.

Me: "Did I tell you that I tend to worry way too much? Bad habit this yoga teacher has! Biking, skiing, and worrying are some of the things I do well."

Clint: "I think you're right. It is a habit, and you can change a habit. Do you want to be a worrier? Or would you like to be something different? What kind of a person doesn't worry?"

Me: "A person that is self-confident, relaxed, and has complete trust that the Universe always brings her exactly what she needs exactly when she needs it."

Clint: "Beautifully put, girl! Write that down and put it on your bathroom mirror. 'I am a self-confident, relaxed person who has complete trust that the Universe always brings me exactly what I need, when I need it.'"

I did write that down and put it in front of my computer, where I spend a good part of each day, and I slowly learned to transform my negative thought pattern into a positive one. Now I help my clients do the same.

What negative thoughts are you telling yourself? How can you flip those around into a positive statement and turn it into your mantra? Write a statement that reminds you that you have the power to replace your self-criticism with self-love instead. Give it a try. It is an extremely powerful, life-transforming exercise.

What to Do When You Can't Change What's Wrong

We've looked at things that can be changed: your mindset, your thoughts, your behaviors... What about things, people, or circumstances that can't be changed? A negative co-worker or boss, an in-law, a parent or sibling, or maybe a challenging situation with your own child?

Perhaps you had a big fight with someone and what's done is done. You can either accept the situation and choose to not let it bother you, or you can develop skills to cope better.

Lucy had three children. One had learning disabilities and was struggling in school. Another had been attacked in the subway and was suffering from PTSD. The third daughter had epilepsy and no combination of medicine seemed to be able to stop the seizures.

All this stress had caused Lucy to turn to food in unhealthy ways, and she gained thirty-five pounds. She was drinking from three to six coffees every morning to try to boost her energy. She was not drinking enough water nor getting enough sleep.

We started by getting her to reduce her coffee and increase her water intake. Her headaches soon disappeared. Then she lost seven pounds by following her body type's plan.

And then she hit a plateau.

Lucy admitted her inner saboteur was rebelling; she didn't want to follow her plan anymore, so she quit for a month and her weight stayed the same.

At this time, she decided to try putting her daughter with epilepsy on a high-fat diet. According to studies reported in the *Lancet Neurology* medical journal, the diet had helped a third of children with epilepsy who had tried it. It was strict. There were many hospital visits for tests to make sure the fat content was appropriate. Everything her daughter ate had to be monitored and any changes had to be charted.

Lucy found a support group for parents of children with epilepsy through the hospital. It was the first time she had ever received any emotional support, and it helped her tremendously. She resumed following her own healthy eating plan more closely. "How can I expect my daughter to follow a strict plan if I can't follow mine?" she said. "I have to set an example."

Over time, her weight continued to decrease. At one session, she told me in tears that the high-fat diet was not working for her daughter. She had long had a dream that her daughter would be cured and lead a normal life. After the few months we had been working together, she was heartbroken to finally accept this might never happen. Working through her emotions and finally coming to terms with her daughter's disability, Lucy was able to stop using food to suppress her fear and disappointment. As a result, she lost thirty-seven pounds and then maintained the healthier weight.

It takes time and effort, but with some good support, we can come to terms with seemingly insurmountable situations. Perhaps you can find a support group or at least some friends who can help you with a problem that's not going away.

Maintaining Healthy Habits

When I read a book or take a course, I'm always excited to implement everything I've learned. Over time, the excitement wanes and that new positive resolve can fall by the wayside. Here are a few suggestions to help you stay on track long term.

Don't Be Overly Hard on Yourself

We all have an inner saboteur. Based on my own experience and that of my numerous clients, that nagging internal voice will often exclaim:

"You will never do this! So why even try?"

"You're just going to fail again. How many times have you already tried?"

"Just have one piece. How could it possibly hurt? It'll make you feel better."

"You can start again on Monday... Or the beginning of next month..."

The internal saboteur has likely been driving your bus for a long time. It's time to take back the steering wheel. One of my clients who had a shy demeanor surprised me by saying she was throwing her inner saboteur under the bus!

My clients often start off their weekly sessions by telling me all the things that they did "wrong" or "failed" to do. I remind them about what they have done right, how many changes that they *have* instilled. They often forget how much they have done, how far they've come.

This is where journaling your progress can be of help. Also, taking time out to look back on each week and jotting down a few notes about what went *right*.

It's so easy to fall into the trap of feeling we're not doing enough, not good enough. I think everyone, from the administrative assistant to the CEO of a multimillion-dollar corporation, is plagued by self-doubt at times.

I've long struggled with my inner saboteur, putting me down, calling me names like stupid, telling me I was not doing enough, not good enough, causing me to feel ashamed for never having married or not driving a nicer car.

When I first joined a gym many years ago, I felt intimidated by all the machines. I had no idea how they worked. I was worried about being observed and judged. On my third day there, I tripped over a wooden box and badly scraped my shin. A few days later when my massage therapist saw the wound, she asked me what happened.

"I'm so stupid; I tripped at the gym," I blurted out.

"Sue-Anne, listen to your words..." she replied. "It was an accident."

A lightbulb went off in my head. I realized how right she was. From that point onward, I rarely, if ever, allowed my inner saboteur to call me names aloud. That inner saboteur still occasionally slips into an internal derogatory thought now and then, but I am more mindful of being kind to myself. Practising mindfulness — which is just being more aware of what you are thinking and doing in each moment as much as possible — is key to catching your inner saboteur. Pay attention to that inner voice. Stop it when it starts repeating itself. Prove it wrong.

Ask your partner or a good friend to point out if they ever hear that inner saboteur putting you down or canceling your joy out loud. Replace those thoughts with positive statements. Keep focusing on your positive qualities and what is going well as you continue to work on yourself.

Learn to Respond to a Situation, Rather than React to It

You may use unhealthy food as a reward, or you may reach for an unhealthy snack when you have a knee-jerk reaction to an unpleasant event. By practising mindfulness, you can pause before saying or doing anything.

Start by identifying your feelings: "Okay, here is a situation that is causing me to feel _____." Then take a step back and choose your response: "I am recognizing (this event) for what it is, and I am aware of my response. This time I am going to try to choose a different method of coping, rather than slipping into an old pattern."

Each time you take a minute to check in with yourself and your thoughts, you improve at learning how to transform your stressors into opportunities for growth and finding healthier ways to celebrate your wins.

My client Norma practised catching herself before eating unhealthy snacks.

"I'm pausing for that split second and realizing how having those chips or cookie will make me feel awful for the rest of the afternoon. And not only physically, but mentally. If I have those chips or cookie, then I start beating myself up and it doesn't stop. I don't want to feel that way anymore," she said.

Working with her new thinking habit, she dropped 20 pounds in 10 weeks.

It's key to begin seeing junk food as something that will ultimately cause pain rather than pleasure. Rather than focusing on the initial 'hit', picture how you feel afterward.

When I eat something that's not good for me, my digestive system has a hard time with it and I invariably don't sleep well.

When I eat healthily, I feel great and have tons of energy. That's a life-changing 'hit' that brings true pleasure day after day.

Use Mindfulness to Overcome Old Patterns

Mindfulness is essential to healthy eating. When we eat mindlessly, we tend to eat too fast and too much.

Get rid of distractions while you eat. Put away all TV, computer, and phone screens. Share your meals with your family and friends instead. Or, if you are on your own, cut out all distractions, slow down, and take a few deep breaths to center yourself. Focus on the food, enjoying the textures, flavors, chewing slowly and appreciating every bite.

Janet practised mindfulness to overcome her sweet cravings.

"I found out that overeating and my abuse of sugar is about not valuing myself," she said. "I don't think people really understand that nutrition and emotional eating are connected. I didn't. It's a powerful revelation."

Janet also learned that the urge to engage in emotional eating is valuable information — when she gets the urge, she knows there is something else going on. It's time to slow down and pay attention to what she's feeling.

"The biggest aha for me is that cravings pass, and I don't have to answer the door when they ring my bell!"

Find Other Ways to Celebrate

The food industry tends to market unhealthy foods as a pleasurable way to reward ourselves. Don't be fooled!

When you eat crap, you feel like crap.

The more you eat healthy, nourishing food, the less your body will desire and tolerate unhealthy food.

In his book *Atomic Habits*, James Clear suggests that when you want to reward yourself, ask: "What would a healthy person do?"

If you keep on asking that question, you will become that healthy person.

Find other ways to reward yourself other than food. Allow yourself some time to do an activity you enjoy. Treat yourself to a massage or some new clothes.

Hey, Your Body is Talking to You!

Your body knows what is good for you. Pay attention to all the messages it is sending you. How do you feel when you wake up in the morning? Are you getting enough sleep? How do you feel when you eat certain foods? How are you managing your stress? Are you setting healthy boundaries and saying no when you need? Do you sit in front of the TV or laptop every night absorbing negative information? Do you end up in front of the fridge or pantry when you're overtired?

I encourage you to find ways to nurture and nourish your body, soul, and mind with things that you love. Eat good food in moderation. And bring other enjoyable things into your life: relaxing music, exercise, motivational reading, hobbies, journaling, calling or getting together with supportive friends.

This journey is about far more than weight loss, as Louise Hay said, "When we create peace and harmony and balance in our minds, we will find it in our lives."

Part Four

Recipes for Each Body Type

E arly in my practice, I created a cookbook for my clients called *High on Health, Low on Sugar*. I've chosen five recipes best suited for each body type from that book to share here.

Recipe Index

Recipes for the Gonad Type

Recipes for the Thyroid Type

Recipes for the Adrenal Type

Recipes for the Pituitary Type

Recipes for the Gonad Type

The Gonad Type tends to be very busy with family and work. My selected recipes are simple, fast, and delicious meals that the whole family will love.

Creamy Italian Dressing
Makes 2½ cups

This healthy dressing is delicious and helps satisfy cravings for creamy dishes.

    ½ pound soft tofu, crumbled
    ½ cup water
    ½ cup extra virgin olive oil
    ⅓ cup unpasteurized red wine vinegar
    1 tablespoon Dijon mustard
    1 teaspoon dried basil
    1 teaspoon dried oregano
    ½ small red onion
    1 garlic clove, peeled
    1 teaspoon salt

Place all the ingredients into a blender and mix until smooth. The dressing stores well in the refrigerator for 4 to 5 days. It's great with cold pasta salad.

Fast and Easy Sauce for Pasta or a Stir Fry

Makes 2 servings

I make this when I'm hungry and in a hurry. You can just throw the ingredients into a pan without measuring them exactly, using larger quantities for larger amounts of pasta or stir-fry vegetables. Adjust the suggested amounts to your needs and taste.

1 tablespoon extra-virgin olive oil
½ onion, sliced
2 cloves of garlic, minced
Optional: 1 tablespoon fresh ginger, minced
2 tablespoons tahini (which is a sesame butter or sesame paste)
2 tablespoons Bragg Liquid Aminos
Seasoning of your choice (Dried basil, oregano, or other herbs)
3 to 4 tablespoons water

For a pasta dish: Cook the pasta of your choice separately as directed. Warm the oil in a frying pan over medium heat. Sauté the onions and garlic until soft. Add the tahini, Bragg Liquid Aminos and water and stir until slightly thickened. Use more water if necessary. Add the strained pasta and stir to coat it completely.

For a stir fry: Sauté the onion, garlic, and minced ginger. Add and sauté the other vegetables of your choice to the desired tenderness. Add the tahini, Bragg Liquid Aminos and water to form the sauce. Serve over brown rice or pasta.

Mexican Rice and Bean Casserole
Serves 6

This easy-to-prepare, gratifying dish is a big hit with adults and kids!

½ cup water
1 onion, chopped
2 cloves garlic, minced
1½ cups mushrooms, chopped
2 red or green peppers, chopped
¾ cup long-grain brown rice
2 cups cooked red kidney beans or 1 can (19 oz/540 ml), rinsed
1 can tomatoes (28 oz/796 ml)
1 tablespoon chili powder
2 teaspoons cumin
¼ teaspoon cayenne
1 cup shredded low-fat mozzarella cheese

Preheat oven to 350° F. In a large skillet or Dutch oven, heat the water over low heat. Add the onion, garlic, mushrooms, and bell peppers; simmer, stirring often, until the onion is tender, about 10 minutes. Add the rice, beans, tomatoes, chili powder, cumin and cayenne. Cover and simmer until the rice is tender and most of the liquid is absorbed, which is about 45 minutes. Transfer to a baking dish and sprinkle with the cheese. Bake for 15 minutes.

Sweet Potato and Coconut Milk Soup

Serves 6

This soup is always a big hit because of the interesting mix of flavors. For a milder version, use a little less chili and cayenne.

5 cups vegetable stock or water
2 large (4 cups) sweet potatoes, diced
1 large Spanish onion, diced
1 medium stalk of celery, diced
1 medium carrot, diced
1 large clove of garlic, minced
1 tablespoon fresh ginger, minced
1 large bay leaf
1 teaspoon sea salt
1 teaspoon ground coriander
1 teaspoon cumin
1 teaspoon dried oregano
¼ - ½ teaspoon crushed dried chili, or to taste
¼ teaspoon cayenne, or to taste
Optional: ¼ cup cilantro roots, minced
1 can (13.5 oz/ 400 ml) coconut milk
1-2 tablespoons Bragg Liquid Aminos, or to taste
¼ cup cilantro leaves as a topping

Bring the 5 cups of vegetable stock (or water) with the vegetables to a boil in a three-quart pot over medium-high heat. Add the garlic, ginger, bay leaf, sea salt, herbs, and spices. Add the cilantro roots. Turn the heat to low and simmer for 15 minutes. Purée the soup in a food processor or blender with the coconut milk and Bragg Liquid Aminos soy sauce. Return the soup to the pot. Simmer for 5 minutes. Adjust the seasonings to your taste. Serve topped with the cilantro greens.

Three Bean Salad

Serves 6

Easy to make, colorful and tasty, this bean salad is perfect for picnics or potlucks.

2 cups green beans
2 cups yellow beans
2 cups cooked kidney beans or 1 can (19 oz/540 ml), rinsed
¼ cup chopped green onions or thinly sliced onion
¼ to ½ cup diced red pepper
⅓ cup apple cider vinegar (unpasteurized)
¼ cup first cold-pressed safflower or canola oil
½ teaspoon sea salt
A dash of freshly ground pepper
1 large clove of garlic, minced

Chop and steam the green and yellow beans in a steamer basket over boiling water. Transfer to a bowl and allow to cool. Add the kidney beans, red pepper, and green onions (or sliced onion). Combine the ingredients for the dressing. Pour the dressing over the beans. Toss well. Cover and refrigerate for three hours or overnight, tossing occasionally.

Recipes for the Thyroid Type

Thyroid Types do best with a lot of protein, starting at breakfast to help reduce cravings for sweets or carbs later in the day. These are some of my favorite high-protein recipes.

Carrot Raisin Oatmeal Power Bars

Makes approximately 12- 16 bars

I have given this recipe to literally hundreds of people, including most every client, numerous friends, cycling buddies, and conference attendees. These bars are delicious, filling snacks and so much healthier than packaged sugary granola bars. They provide a satisfying mid-afternoon snack that keeps your blood sugar balanced and your energy steady until dinnertime.

1½ cups spelt or Kamut Khorasan wheat flour
1½ cups rolled oats
1 tablespoon cinnamon
½ teaspoon allspice
½ teaspoon sea salt
½ cup + 2 tablespoons maple syrup
12 drops liquid stevia
½ cup organic first cold-pressed canola oil
½ cup tahini (sesame butter)
1 tablespoon fresh ginger, grated
1 cup carrots, finely grated
1 cup raisins
1 cup chopped walnuts

Preheat oven to 350° F. Combine the first five dry ingredients in a large bowl. Mix the next seven wet ingredients in a separate bowl. Add the wet ingredients to the dry ingredients and mix well so no lumps of flour remain. Fold in the carrots, raisins, and walnuts evenly. Grease an 8x8-inch baking dish (or one that is slightly bigger) with some butter or oil. Scrape all the batter from the bowl into the baking dish and smooth out the top to make the batter even. Bake for 30 to 40 minutes or until golden brown. Cool to room temperature for one hour before slicing into bars. Wrap individually. They freeze well.

Deviled Tofu
Serves 4

This mock 'egg salad' is a sumptuous spread for sandwiches or as a source of protein alongside a vegetable salad.

(1 lb/454 grams) organic firm tofu
¼ to ½ cup mayonnaise (real or tofu-based)
¼ teaspoon coriander
⅛ teaspoon cumin
½ teaspoon curry
¼ teaspoon salt
⅛ teaspoon paprika
A dash of garlic powder
¼ teaspoon Bragg Liquid Aminos
1 tablespoon Dijon mustard (or less to taste)
¼ cup green relish
¼ cup (or more) celery, diced

Squeeze the excess water from the tofu by wrapping it in a clean dish towel and pressing on it. Then crumble the tofu using a food processor. Transfer the crumbled tofu to a bowl. Add the other ingredients and mix thoroughly.

Ginger Marmalade Chicken

Serves 4 to 6

Another simple dish that will have people asking for the recipe.

> 4 to 6 skinless chicken breasts (depending on their size)
> ½ cup marmalade
> 2 teaspoons Dijon mustard
> 1 tablespoon Bragg Liquid Aminos
> 2 tablespoons natural rice vinegar
> 1 tablespoon fresh ginger, chopped

For the sauce:

> ½ to 1 tablespoon cornstarch
> 1 tablespoon water

Preheat oven to 400° F. Place the chicken breasts in a baking dish. In a bowl, combine the marmalade, Dijon mustard, Bragg Liquid Aminos, vinegar and ginger until well mixed. Spoon it evenly over the chicken breasts. Bake for 20 to 25 minutes, until the chicken is cooked through and golden brown on top.

Sauce: Pour the liquid from the baking dish into a small pot and set over a medium heat. Mix the cornstarch with 1 tablespoon of water in a mug and add it to the saucepan. Heat and stir until thickened. Serve each chicken breast with some of the hot marmalade sauce.

Maple-Ginger Tofu (or Chicken or Salmon)
Makes 4 servings

I often make this with salmon. The ginger and toasted sesame oil are a delicious combination.

Pick your protein:

1 - 1½ pounds firm or extra firm tofu, rinsed and sliced into cutlets or triangles
1 pound organic skinless, boneless chicken breasts
1 pound organically raised or wild-caught salmon

Sauce:

3 tablespoons Bragg Liquid Aminos
3 tablespoons ginger, minced (or less to taste)
¼ cup maple syrup
1 tablespoon brown rice vinegar
1 teaspoon toasted sesame oil
1 to 2 cloves of garlic, minced (or less to taste)
Optional: fresh chives, cilantro or parsley

Combine sauce ingredients in a bowl.

For the tofu or chicken dish: Heat a skillet to a medium-high temperature. Add the oil and let it heat up. Place the tofu or chicken in the skillet and sear both sides. Switch the burner to a low temperature and add the sauce. Cover and simmer until the sauce caramelizes. Top with fresh herbs.

For the salmon: Preheat the oven to 375° F. Heat a skillet to a medium-high temperature. Add the oil and let it heat up. Sear the fish on both sides. Place the salmon in a baking pan (ceramic, if you have one, as it evenly distributes heat) and pour the sauce over the fish. Bake for about 10 minutes or until the salmon is cooked to your liking. Garnish with fresh herbs and serve.

Stacey's Keep-You-Going Protein Pancakes
Serves 2

My friend Stacey created these protein-packed pancakes when her daughters were competing in gymnastics. They go well with fresh chunks of apple or berries.

½ cup oatmeal
½ cup of 1% cottage cheese (preferably low-sodium)
1 whole egg
2 egg whites
1 teaspoon vanilla
1 teaspoon coconut oil (for frying)

Blend all the ingredients, except the coconut oil, in a food processor or mixer. Melt the coconut oil in a skillet over medium heat. Place a generous spoonful or two of the mixture in the skillet for each pancake, depending on the size you want, making sure to keep a bit of distance between them. Fry until golden brown on both sides.

Trail Mix
Makes 12 servings

This is one of my go-to snacks, highly nutrient dense and filling. Perfect as an afternoon snack for Thyroid Types and ideal for traveling as it keeps well.

½ cup raw almonds
½ cup walnuts
½ cup pumpkin seeds
½ cup sunflower seeds
½ cup raisins
½ cup dried apricots

Mix together in a bowl and store in a large glass jar.

Recipes for the Adrenal Type

Adrenal Types love savory dishes, especially with a healthy gravy that adds flavor. I've chosen savoury recipes and healthy recipes that will keep the Adrenal Type satisfied.

Garden Veggie Antipasto

A perfect way to get more veggies into your day, as a delicious snack or side dish

   1 small cauliflower, cut in florets
   ½ bunch broccoli, trimmed and cut into florets
   3 medium carrots, cut into sticks
   1/3 cup unpasteurized red wine vinegar
   ¼ cup extra virgin olive oil
   1 teaspoon basil
   1 teaspoon oregano
   1 teaspoon thyme
   1 garlic clove minced
   ½ teaspoon sundried sea salt
   Freshly ground pepper to taste

Put water in large saucepan with steamer basket, bring to a boil. Put the vegetables into the steamer basket, cover and steam about 5 minutes. (Or a little longer, you want them crunchy, do not overcook) Put the veggies in a bowl.

Put the vinaigrette ingredients in a jar, cover with the lid and shake.

Pour the vinaigrette over the steamed vegetables. Toss until well coated. Refrigerate at least 30 minutes before serving.

Hearty Vegetable Soup
Serves 6

This richly flavored, Spanish-style soup is almost like a stew, and just as filling and delicious. The vegetables in this soup can be combined with any other green vegetable. Carrots, pumpkin or squash can replace the sweet potato.

1 tablespoon olive oil
1 cup chopped onion
3 medium garlic cloves, crushed
1 stalk celery, minced
2 cups peeled, diced sweet potato
1 teaspoon salt
2 teaspoons mild paprika
1 teaspoon turmeric
1 teaspoon basil
A dash of cinnamon
A dash of cayenne
1 bay leaf
3 cups vegetable stock or water
2 medium ripe size tomatoes, diced, or 1 cup of canned diced tomatoes
1 medium red bell pepper, diced
1½ cups cooked chickpeas or 1 can (14 oz/ 398 ml), drained

Heat the olive oil in a large pot. Add the onion, garlic, celery, and sweet potato and sauté over medium heat for about 5 minutes. Add seasonings and water.

Cover and simmer about 15 minutes. Add the tomatoes, bell pepper and chickpeas. Cover and simmer for about 10 minutes, or until all the vegetables are as tender as you like them. Taste to adjust seasonings and serve.

Homemade Ketchup

Makes 8 servings

Regular ketchup is so high in sugar. Here is an easy, sugar-free ketchup that's tasty and low in salt.

  1 - 12 oz. can salt-free tomato paste
  ½ cup unpasteurized apple cider vinegar
  ½ cup water
  ½ teaspoon sun-dried sea salt
  1 teaspoon oregano
  ⅛ teaspoon cumin
  ⅛ teaspoon nutmeg
  ⅛ teaspoon pepper
  ½ teaspoon mustard powder
  A squeeze of garlic from press (or a dash of garlic powder)

Mix all the ingredients together. Store in a jar in the fridge.

Hot Tamale Pie
Makes one 8-inch square pie

This is a real crowd pleaser. Made with beans, lots of vegetables and spices, and a cornmeal crust, it has an enticingly different flavor combination. The pie keeps well in the refrigerator for up to five days. Just reheat in the oven at 325 - 350° F for about 30 minutes and serve. Show off the two colorful layers by baking it in a glass dish if you have one.

> 1 tablespoon extra virgin olive oil
> 1 medium onion, finely chopped
> 1 medium yellow, red or green bell pepper, seeded and finely chopped
> 2 garlic cloves, minced
> 1 can (16 oz/473 ml) unsweetened tomato sauce
> 1 can (16 oz/473 ml) pinto beans, rinsed and drained
> 1 ear of corn, kernels cut off the cob, or ¾ cup of frozen corn that has been thawed
> 1 teaspoon chili powder
> 1 teaspoon ground cumin
> 1 teaspoon fine sea salt
> A pinch of cayenne pepper
> 3 cups water
> 1 cup yellow stone-ground cornmeal
> 1 tablespoon lemon juice
> 1 teaspoon Dijon mustard
> Another ½ teaspoon fine sea salt

Preheat oven to 350° F. Heat the olive oil in a large frying pan over medium-high heat. Add the onion, bell pepper and garlic and cook until softened, about 6 to 8 minutes. Remove from heat and stir in the tomato sauce, pinto beans, corn, chili powder, cumin, salt, and cayenne. Pour into an 8x8-inch glass baking dish. Boil the water in a large saucepan, add the cornmeal, lemon juice, mustard, and salt.

Stir until mixed. Bring to a boil over medium-high heat. Immediately reduce the heat to low and simmer, stirring often, until thickened, about 3 to 5 minutes. Spread the cooked cornmeal over the bean mixture. Bake for 30 minutes. Cool for 10 minutes before serving.

Hummus
Makes 1 ½ cups

Whenever I bring this to a potluck, everyone is surprised that I make my own as they are used to store-bought. They all rave about it, as this tastes so much better. I timed myself to see how fast and easy it is to make. It took me four minutes.

>   2 cups chickpeas
>   1/3 cup tahini (sesame butter)
>   1 or 2 medium garlic cloves, chopped
>   1 teaspoon basil
>   ½ teaspoon salt
>   ½ teaspoon cumin
>   ¼ to ½ cup water

Place everything in a food processor and blend. Add water gradually to desired consistency.

Savory Vegan Gravy

Makes 1 ¼ cups

No need to have a roast to make this gravy! This is easy and delicious poured on top of vegetarian fare, meat, grains and other food.

  2 tablespoons extra virgin olive oil
  2 tablespoons Kamut Khorasan wheat or spelt flour
  1 cup hot water
  2 tablespoons Bragg Liquid Aminos
  ¼ teaspoon dried basil
  Optional: sliced onions or mushrooms

Heat the oil in a frying pan. Sauté onions or mushrooms until soft. Add the flour, stirring to remove all lumps. Slowly pour in the hot water, stirring briskly with a whisk to ensure no lumps. Add in the Bragg Liquid Aminos and basil. Stir and allow the gravy to thicken.

Veggie Pâté
Makes 8 servings

This pâté smells heavenly when baking, and it tastes great! I use an 8x8-inch pan so that it isn't too thick and cooks thoroughly. A food processor will save you prep time. You can buy nutritional yeast at any natural food store. Usually sold in bulk, it has a tangy, almost cheesy flavor. It is also good sprinkled on salads and provides the vitamin B12 that vegetarians are often lacking.

⅓ cup old-fashioned oats
½ cup sunflower seeds
1 clove garlic
2 onions
1 carrot
1 stalk celery
1 potato
2 tablespoons fresh lemon juice
⅓ cup first cold-pressed organic canola oil
3 tablespoons Bragg Liquid Aminos
¾ cup Spelt or Kamut Khorasan wheat flour
1 teaspoon dried basil
½ teaspoon dried thyme
¼ teaspoon dried sage
½ cup hot water
⅔ cup nutritional yeast

Preheat the oven to 350° F. Grind the oats and seeds in a food processor. Transfer them to a bowl. Chop the vegetables into large chunks and pulse them in the food processor into tiny pieces. Add them to the bowl and mix in all the remaining ingredients. Transfer the bowl's contents to a baking dish. Bake for 1 hour. Cool and transfer to a plate.

Recipes for the Pituitary Type

Pituitary Types do well with a lot of protein. I've chosen healthy recipes with beans that are high in protein. Here are some colorful, delicious meals that are both satisfying and particularly nourishing for your body type.

Apricot Chicken Divine

The sauce manages to be creamy without cream! It tops this dish to make it both flavorful and healthy.

- 2 tablespoons butter
- 2 tablespoons extra virgin olive oil
- 6 to 8 skinned chicken breast halves
- ½ cup Kamut Khorasan wheat flour
- 1 teaspoon salt
- ⅓ to ½ cup apricot preserves or apricot jam sweetened with grape juice
- 1 tablespoon Dijon mustard
- ½ cup yogurt
- 2 tablespoons slivered almonds

Preheat oven to 375° F. Melt butter with oil in a shallow baking pan. Meanwhile, shake the chicken in a plastic bag filled with the flour and salt until the chicken is coated. Place the chicken in a single layer in the baking pan and bake for 25 minutes. Combine the apricot preserves (or jam), mustard, and yogurt. Spread the apricot mixture on the chicken and bake until done, about 20 to 30 minutes. Just before serving, brown the slivered almonds lightly in an oven. Sprinkle the almonds over the chicken and serve it over brown rice.

Black Bean and Corn Salad
Serves 8

This dish serves up a bowl of beautiful colors and everyone loves the fresh lime taste. It's a big hit at potlucks. The salad can be prepared a few hours ahead, but don't add the avocado until serving time.

⅓ cup freshly squeezed lime juice
½ cup extra virgin olive oil
1 garlic clove, minced
1 teaspoon fine sea salt
⅛ teaspoon cayenne pepper
2 (15 oz / 443 ml) cans black beans, rinsed and drained or 4 cups cooked black beans
2 ears of corn with kernels cut off the cob, or 1½ cups frozen organic corn (thawed)
1 avocado peeled and cut into ½-inch pieces
1 small red pepper, seeded and cut into ½-inch pieces
2 medium tomatoes cut into ½-inch pieces
6 green onions, with green tops, finely chopped
1 fresh hot chili pepper or less, seeded and minced
½ cup fresh cilantro, coarsely chopped

Put the lime juice, olive oil, garlic, salt, and cayenne in a small jar with a tight-fitting lid. Cover the jar with its lid and shake until the ingredients are well mixed. In a salad bowl, combine the beans, corn, avocado, bell pepper, tomatoes, green onions, chili pepper, and cilantro. Shake the lime dressing and pour it over the salad. Stir until well coated. Refrigerate and adjust the seasonings before serving.

Minestrone Soup
Serves 8

Full of vegetables and noodles, this hearty Italian soup is a meal all by itself. A little low-fat cheese grated on top is a nice touch. Garlic bread goes well with it, too.

2 cups Kamut Khorasan wheat shell macaroni or other or whole grain pasta (penne or fusilli)
1 tablespoon extra virgin olive oil
1 medium onion, chopped
1 medium carrot, chopped
1 medium celery stalk with leaves, chopped
4 garlic cloves, minced
8 cups vegetable stock
3 medium tomatoes, finely chopped, or 1 (14 oz/398 ml) can unsweetened Italian tomatoes, undrained, chopped
2 cups cooked or canned kidney beans, drained
1 medium potato, unpeeled, cut into ½-inch pieces
½ teaspoon dried rosemary
2 teaspoons dried basil
1 teaspoon dried oregano
1 bay leaf
½ teaspoon fine sea salt
¼ teaspoon freshly ground black pepper
Optional: 3 cups (about ½ of a small head) finely shredded green cabbage
½ cup fresh parsley, finely chopped

In a medium pot of lightly salted boiling water, cook the noodles until just tender, about 6 minutes. Drain, rinse under cold water and drain again. Set the noodles aside. In a large pot, heat the olive oil over medium heat. Add the onion, carrot, celery, and garlic. Cook, stirring occasionally until softened, about 5 minutes. Stir in vegetable stock, tomatoes, potato, beans, rosemary, basil, oregano, bay leaf, salt, and pepper. Bring to a simmer and cook, partially covered, until the tomatoes are almost tender, about 8 minutes. Grate a little low-fat mozzarella or other cheese on top if you like.

Salmon Cakes

Makes four large cakes.

These delicious salmon cakes are quick and easy to make.

1 (7.5 oz/213 ml) can wild-caught salmon (or cooked salmon)
1 medium sweet potato
1 egg
2 tablespoons brown rice flour or Kamut Khorasan wheat or other whole grain flour
2 scallions, chopped
1 stalk celery, chopped
2 tablespoons extra virgin olive oil
½ teaspoon sea salt
A pinch of paprika

Preheat the oven to 350° F. Steam the sweet potato until soft. Drain the canned salmon. Using a fork, combine and mash together all the ingredients into a bowl. Separate into four patties and place on a lightly oiled baking tray. Bake until golden, about 45 minutes. Alternatively, they can be fried in a little oil over medium heat until golden brown on both sides.

Vegan Lentil 'Meatballs'
Makes approximately 20 lentil 'meatballs'

These round nuggets taste great with or without sauce. For a softer, more traditional type of 'meatball,' use your favorite marinara or pasta sauce. They can also be air-fried and served alone for a crunchier, more textured appetizer or meal element. What's also great is that these freeze well before or after cooking.

  1 tablespoon olive oil
  1 yellow onion, finely chopped
  1 large carrot, peeled and diced
  4 cloves garlic, minced
  1 cup pumpkin seeds
  2 cups cooked green lentils (approximately ¾ cup when dry) or 2 cups canned lentils, drained
  2 tablespoons tomato paste
  1 teaspoon dried oregano
  1 teaspoon dried basil
  ¼ cup nutritional yeast
  1 teaspoon sea salt

Preheat oven to 400° F. Sauté the onion, carrot, and garlic in a skillet with the oil until softened, about 5 minutes. Line a large baking tray with parchment paper. Pulse the pumpkin seeds in the food processor to break them down. Add the cooked vegetables, cooked lentils, tomato paste and all the seasonings. Combine well, but stop short of turning everything into a purée. Scrape down the sides to fully combine, if required. Taste the mixture and add more seasoning if you'd like. Form the mixture into small balls (approximately 1- to 1½-inch in diameter) and place them on the lined baking sheet. Bake for 25-30 minutes, until golden brown.

Quinoa Tabouleh

Serves 6

I've made this healthy, tasty dish many times. Perfect summer fare. In the winter, I often replace the cucumber with red pepper. It is a real crowd pleaser.

1 cup quinoa
2 cups water
2 medium tomatoes, cut into ½-inch cubes
1 medium cucumber, cut into ½-inch cubes
6 green onions, with tops, finely chopped
1 small red or green bell pepper, seeded and cut into ½-inch cubes
1 cup chopped fresh parsley (I add more)
½ cup finely chopped fresh mint

Dressing:

⅓ cup freshly squeezed lemon juice
⅓ cup extra virgin olive oil
1 garlic clove, minced
1 teaspoon sun-dried sea salt
A pinch, or up to 1/8 teaspoon, cayenne pepper

Put the quinoa in a wire strainer and rinse with hot water. In a medium saucepan, bring the water and the quinoa to a boil over high heat. Reduce the heat to low, cover and simmer 15 minutes or longer until all the water has evaporated. Transfer the quinoa to a bowl and cool completely. Then stir the tomatoes, green onions, cucumber, bell pepper, parsley and mint into the cooled quinoa.

In a small bowl, whisk together the lemon juice, oil, garlic, salt and cayenne pepper. Pour over the quinoa and toss well. Cover and refrigerate for at least 30 minutes before serving.

Acknowledgments

I am first and foremost eternally grateful to all the clients who have believed in me and my approach to eating more healthily for our body type. From those early days when I held my initial consultations in my home office and ran workshops in my living room, you have confirmed for me over many years what you found really worked well and what didn't. This has truly helped me to fine-tune the Bodytypology process. Thank you for putting your trust in me. It has been an honour to create this content with you in mind.

My thanks also go to Julie Gedeon, whose fastidious editing, wonderful suggestions, enthusiasm, and encouragement were instrumental in taking me from writer to author. I also thank the fabulous group in her Writers' Kitchen who met first in her home and then online during the Covid pandemic. Chantal St-Laurent, Terry Soucy, Odette Quenneville-Lalonde, Valerie Redmond, and Stephanie Azran, you were all a constant source of fun and support while providing me with invaluable feedback during my writing of this book.

I also want to thank my dear friend Angie Gallop whose remarkable editing skills, encouragement and humour have been an invaluable gift in helping me to publish numerous articles and newsletters about healthy eating and living over two decades. You helped turn my pages into a book that fills me with pride.

My appreciation goes as well to Ingrid Hein for her insightful review and editing suggestions.

To Alexa Nazzaro and her publishing team who helped me get this book published.

A big thank-you to all the book's early readers, Laura Lewis Hammond, Shari Mayer Gagné, Ana María Giraldo Ramirez M.D., Debora Must, Jennie Whitaker, Jennifer Walker, Renee Mollitt, Dr. Joanna McDonald, Greg Lee, Arantza Izurrategui, Melanie Cleland and Valerie Provost.

Finally, I give my deepest thanks to Phil, the love of my life, for his unwavering belief and support, and his infinite patience with my up and down Thyroid Type energy.

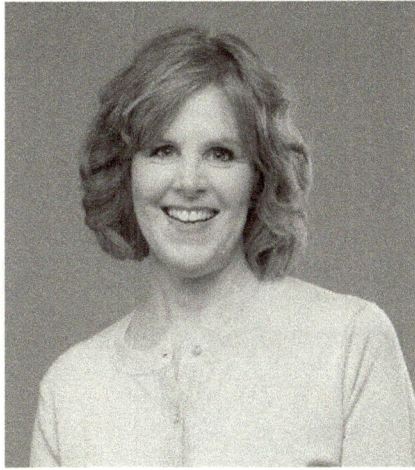

After graduating from Concordia University with a B.A specialization in French/English translation, Sue-Anne Hickey realized that she preferred to work with people rather than a dictionary and thesaurus.

She left for India to train as a yoga teacher. This was part of a year-and-a-half journey around the world. She participated in Vipassana meditation retreats in Thailand and India, studied Tibetan Buddhism and meditation in Nepal, and spent time at Ashrams in India and Bali in search of answers to life's challenges.

Upon her return, Sue-Anne taught yoga and continued learning everything she could about nutrition, taking courses in macrobiotic cooking as well as the Mindfulness Based Stress Management taught by Jon Kabat Zinn.

After years as a yoga teacher, she signed up for naturopath training. Her life changed when she discovered she was a Thyroid Type and needed more protein at breakfast and throughout her day. She couldn't wait to use her newfound knowledge to help others to become healthier.

Sue-Anne combines her Bodytypology eating plan with Rapid Transformational Therapy (R.T.T.), a hypnotherapy modality aimed at identifying and releasing buried, limiting beliefs. The combined approaches have produced a high rate of success in healing emotional eating and other unhealthy habits to promote long-term health, ample energy, and sustained weight loss.

Sue-Anne has written a column on healthier living for her local newspaper and has appeared on the *MindBodyGreen* wellness platform as well as in *Women's World Magazine*. *Bodytypology* is her first book.

Sue-Anne lives with her partner Phil just west of Montreal.

What's Next?

Thank you so much for taking the time to read this book. It's a pleasure to share my passion with you. If you enjoyed *Bodytypology: A System for Optimal Health and Lasting Weight Loss* then you might like read my latest articles and health tips by signing up for my newsletters I send out a few times a week. You can also find free resources such as the Body Type Quiz and Emotional Eating Food Journal at https://www.bodytypology.com/book.html.

Facebook: https://www.facebook.com/4bodytypes/
Instagram: https://www.instagram.com/bodytypology/
YouTube: https://www.youtube.com/@bodytypology

www.ingramcontent.com/pod-product-compliance
Lightning Source LLC
Chambersburg PA
CBHW031126020426
42333CB00012B/245